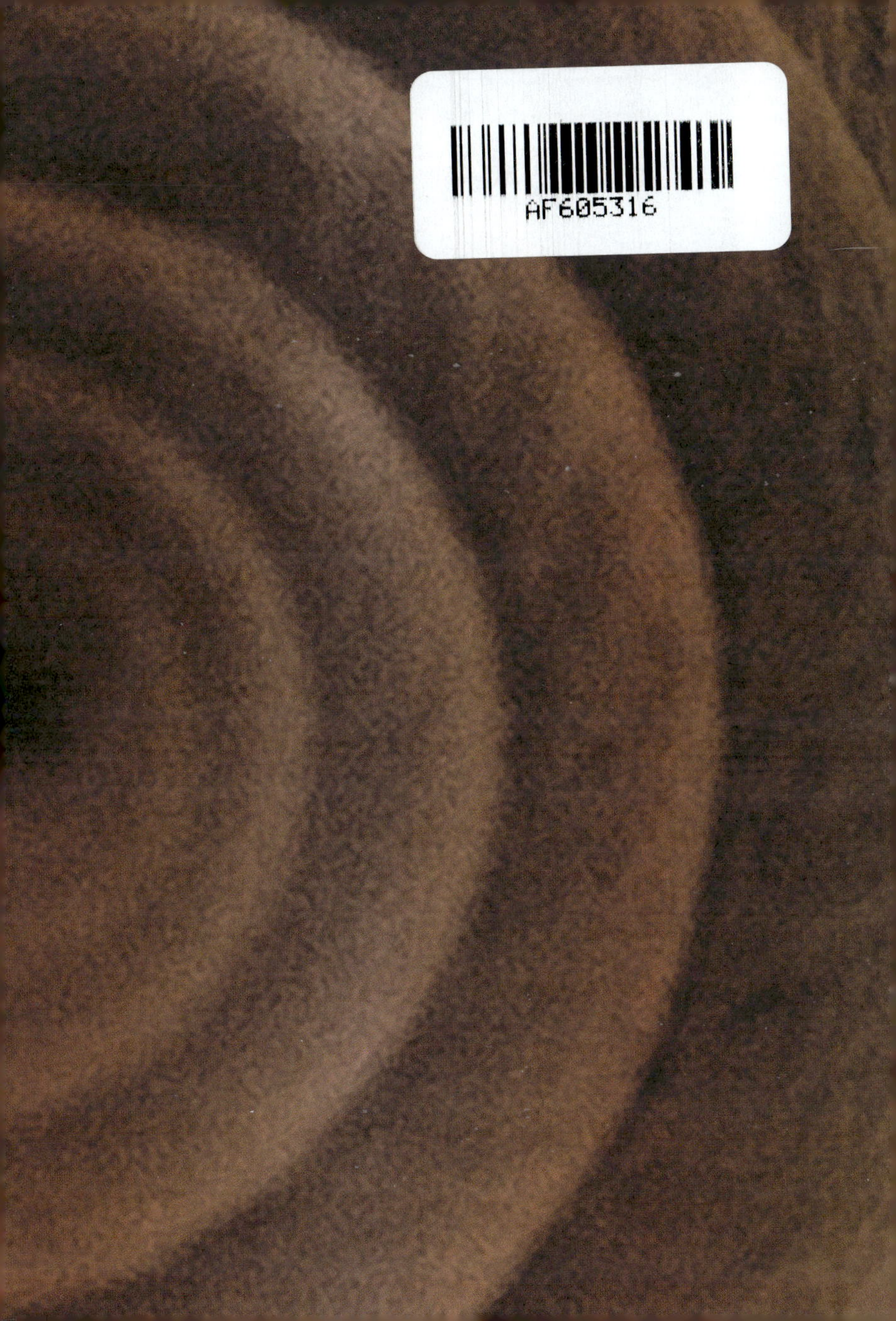

ARA

A Māori guidebook of the mind

ARA

DR HINEMOA ELDER

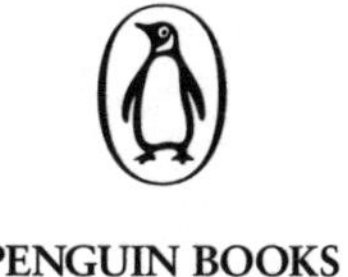

PENGUIN BOOKS

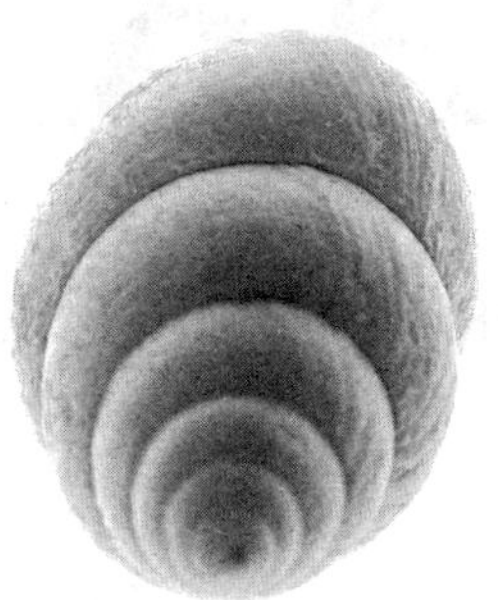

Whakamoemiti ki a Hinengaro

Ka mahara tonu ki a koe, Hinengaro,
E kakama e te huatau, nōu te kakare o ngā wai,
Tēnā tonu te tokerau o te moana.

Tērā te noho i te kāngatungatu,
Tērā te ūkaipō o te whanaungatanga,
Tērā te arero o te kupu.

E hoki rānei te kupu ki te māwhera?
Mā tō aroha ka tukua te kōrero tuku iho
ki ngā mokopuna e piki ake ana, e piki ake ana.

Kei tō huanui te ara ki te oranga,
Kei tō tia te kāpura o te kōingo,
Kei tō tikanga te rangatiratanga.

Ka whakapuaki i tō kupu taurangi ki ahau,
Ka whakaaria mai tēnei whakaau ki ngā reanga,
E haere mai ana, e haere mai ana.

He aha te pononga o te pūpū harakeke?
Anō te kaitiaki o ngā rua.
Anō te hokinga o ngā raumahara.
Anō te painga o Hinengaro.

Atu i te nuku o te whenua, ki te nuku o te moana,
Nei rā tō Hinengaro kāinga.
Ka puta, ka ora, ki te Whaiao, ki te Ao Mārama, e.

NGĀ IHIRANGI

CONTENTS

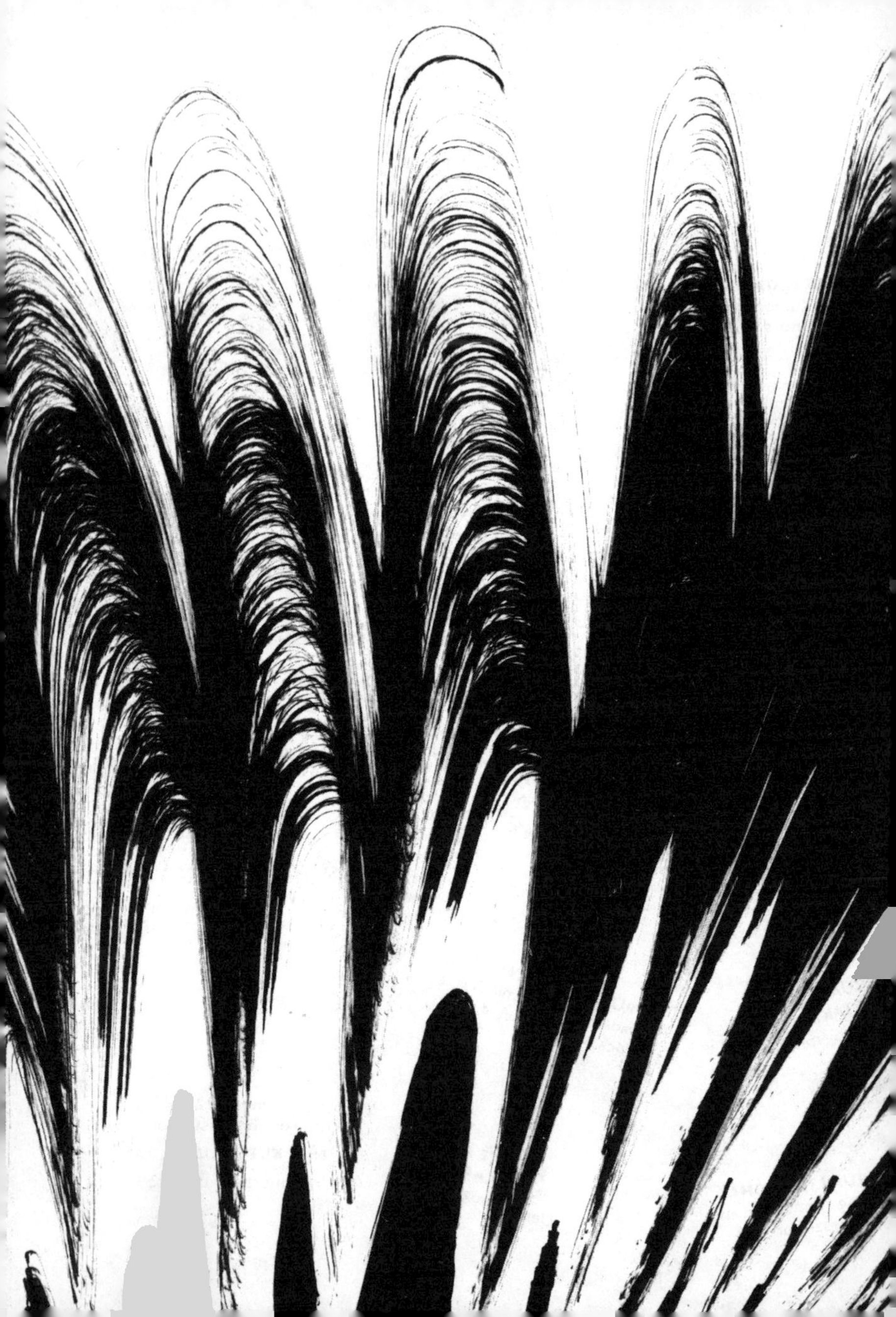

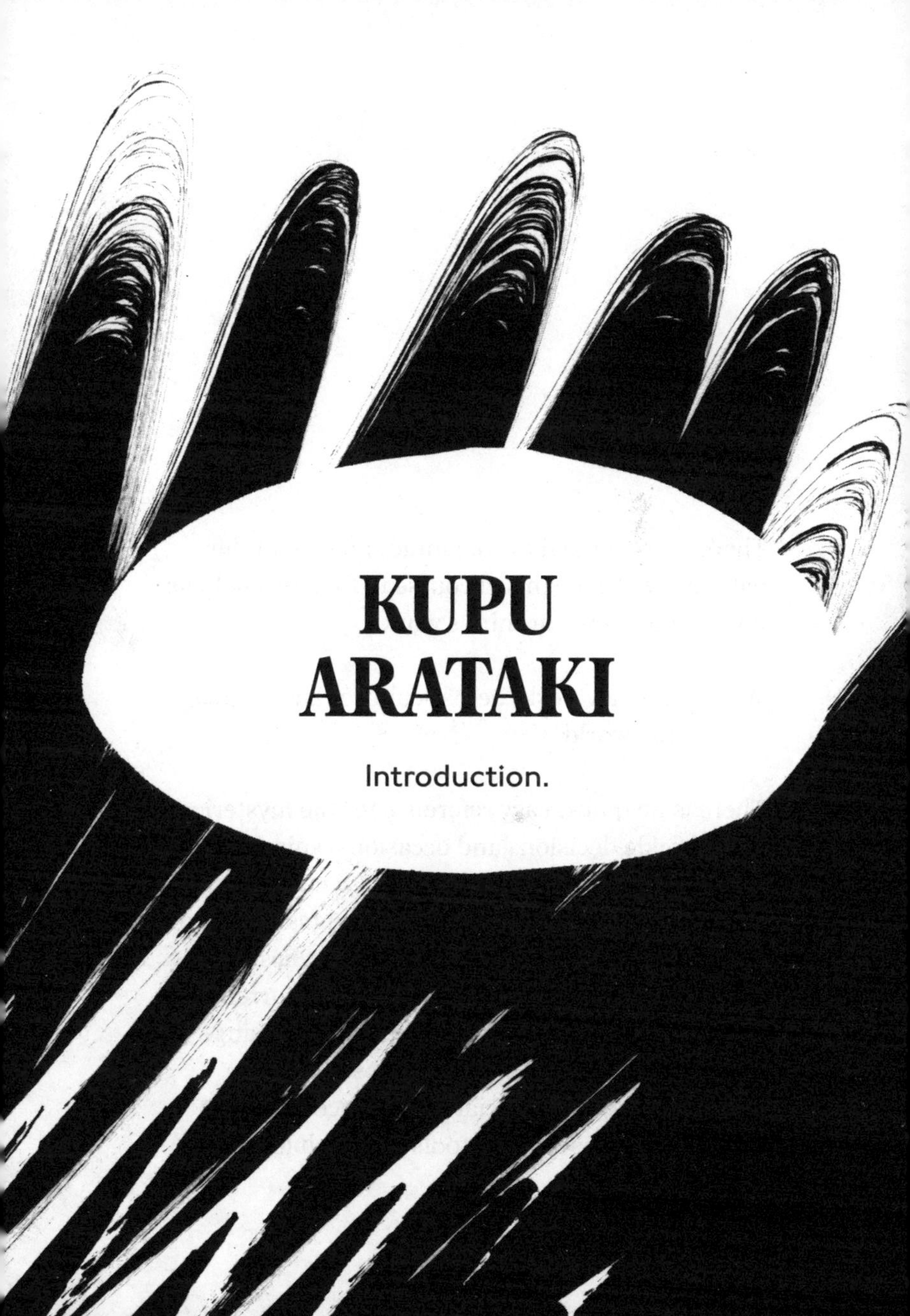

KUPU ARATAKI

Introduction.

There is no manual for the mind; no map of the path, no well-recognised course to follow to help us understand how our minds work.

Well, none that works across cultures and languages around the world.

There is no quick, easy reference for the mysterious mix of fickle decisions and occasional snippets of logic that our minds come up with, our stubborn misplaced beliefs, our tendencies and tastes. There is no one resource that consistently teaches us how to interpret the nature of our thoughts. Current knowledge of neural pathways and the exchange of chemicals still can't explain consciousness. Now in the age of artificial intelligence we might be tempted to use digital tools to search for clues.

But how can we rely on AI to give answers that are accurate, or meaningful? And what happens to our data when we ask our most vulnerable questions about what makes us tick?

Philosophers and scientists have tried to produce such work. Through the ages people have dedicated their lives to developing theories and therapies. Some have fallen out of fashion while others hold sway for a time. Each contributes something useful, and yet all have their flaws.

Thinking about thinking relies on how we are taught and what we learn. And yet we spend so little time critiquing the manner in which this fundamental part of life is formally and informally conveyed.

As a psychiatrist of almost 20 years, a mother, a whānau member, a descendant, I have always been fascinated by the nature of our minds. Wearing these various hats I have witnessed the conflicting ways we engage with activities that involve thinking about thinking. Some approaches emphasise the paramount importance of logic and reason as our examination tools, while emotions are often deemed a lower-order function. The distinction between thinking, feeling and behaviour is often promoted. Some frames of reference focus on our roles in life and how these transition and change across the life span. Others pay attention to how we relive the dynamics of our relationships with our parents.

Whether our lessons occur at home, in school, at work or more generally through the university of our life experiences, we are also taught to have certain expectations of how our minds 'should' work. We learn about priorities that foster autonomy, independence and a sense of individuality. But this perspective doesn't always feel comfortable for those of us who come from cultures which emphasise interdependence, collectivism and reciprocity. This leads to tensions that we might struggle to pinpoint. We might have an uneasy feeling when we are taught to aspire to be separate individuals, in contrast to our life experiences as part of groups, which are essential to who we are.

Increasingly, accelerating and novel pressures in our world, fear and stress in our lives, the voracious appetite for our data, war and conflict, and climate emergency mean we need tools that give us options to think about thinking differently. In that way we can begin to approach the critical challenges we face from perspectives that build cohesive, compassionate decisions and actions.

This book brings forward some of our Māori resources for thinking about thinking. My audacious goal is to provide much-needed life guidance for both our local and global communities.

Throughout medical school and specialist training, I craved examples of our specific Māori ways of thinking about thinking. But what we were taught was heavily influenced by the ideas and theories of people from other parts of the world. These theories have come to exert a huge influence on the therapies that are most commonly offered in mental health services. They hold authority because they have been tested using the most highly valued research designs. Cognitive behavioural theory (CBT), for example, was based on the idea that individuals' interpretations of situations influence their reactions. These interpretations, considered to be 'thoughts', then determined subsequent emotions and actions. This theory identified that our interpretations can be distorted, especially when what the exponents of these ideas called 'psychopathology' is present. The idea was that these patterns of distorted thinking were linked to underlying beliefs that individuals have about themselves, other people, the world and the future. The originators found that when people were provided with therapy based on this theory to change their way of thinking, they felt better and were able to change their behaviour. They also found that this change in their beliefs had some lasting effect.

This work has had a massive influence on current evidence-based interventions for a range of mental health problems worldwide. The many off-shoots of CBT have been manualised, turned into structured sets of tools. These kinds of step-by-step, standardised therapies became part of a cycle of easy-to-repeat studies using randomised controlled trial (RCT) design. This meant that studies testing these kinds of therapies for different conditions lent themselves to replication. Given RCTs are regarded as the highest level of evidence, these therapies took up a dominant position, attracting funding for training and implementation in many health and social services around the world. Developing and delivering manualised training programmes which stuck to these rules became a well-oiled machine.

But like everything, this approach has limitations. For example, CBT does not work so well for those who are practical and hands-on in nature, or those who have a strong collective influence on their core beliefs. For people who prefer to be outdoors rather than sitting and talking about their thoughts, feelings and behaviours, CBT may not be the best fit. Many people of different ages and cultures have their own reasons that make putting their experiences and emotions into words really tough. In my specialty area, child and adolescent psychiatry, the effect size for our patients with depressive illnesses at the end of treatment is around 0.4. That means CBT in this group with this clinical diagnosis has been shown to work 40 per cent of the time when the therapy has finished.* Not a bad result, but it leaves a large group with little or no benefit. The other downside is that you can't easily predict who might respond best to this treatment when you start.

* Cuijpers, P., Karyotaki, E., Ciharova, M., Miguel, C., Noma, H., Stikkelbroek, Y., . . . & Furukawa, T.A. (2023). The effects of psychological treatments of depression in children and adolescents on response, reliable change, and deterioration: A systematic review and meta-analysis. *European child & adolescent psychiatry,* 32(1), 177–192.

What I have learned about these influential ideas and tools is that while they can be useful, they also show that there is room for improvement and the need for other resources.

One of the other aspects that is rarely taught is that the ideas behind cognitive behavioural theories and therapies were based on the work of philosophers from around 2000 years ago. One of these was Epictetus, a Greek. From a young age he stood out as being a brilliant thinker and so was sent to Rome to study. He followed a philosophy known as Stoicism. The Stoics believed that thinking about thinking needed to provide practical help for navigating the challenges of everyday life, to provide guidance for living a life filled with feelings of happiness, tranquillity and a sense of satisfaction. Epictetus theorised that the logic and reasoning parts of the mind's activity helped to settle emotions and behaviours. He summarised these ideas in a book called *Enchiridion*, or 'the manual'. Only sections of his book survive today, but we know it was a best-seller in its day. Roman soldiers carried their own copies everywhere, even into battle.

In one way or another we have been heavily influenced by these concepts from other cultures from another time. Recognising that these ideas from another place persist in dominating current theory and practice has continued to raise questions for me. How can we make space for our Māori constructs of mind in order to ensure our communities have access to our own resources? How could these resources be useful to the world right now, just as those from the Mediterranean have been useful over the past 2000 years? The time is ripe for Indigenous people's ideas and practices to come to the fore. Our ideas have so much to offer given our relationship with Mother Earth and our essential role and ongoing care for the world's remaining biodiversity.

This book is my attempt to create a safe place to explore some aspects of our Māori wellspring of knowledge to help us think about thinking, for global wellbeing.

~

Let me introduce you to our own Māori goddess of the mind, Hinengaro.

She is in charge of everything we think and feel, what we believe and how we see ourselves. She is the one who gives us the tools to make decisions, to grow in our learning. Hinengaro brings us emotions so that we respond with aroha, love in all its forms, with tears, with rage. She has the skills we need to make choices, and to live through the consequences. She drives us to seek out new discoveries beyond what we can comprehend today. She can be restless. She can be calm. Hinengaro can bring her dark shadows and her fears. And she can make colours brighter and music sweeter. Hinengaro is how we conceive of life, death and everything in between. She gives us the knowing of realms beyond the physical — the fantastical, the strange and wondrous. Hers are the creative powers of invention. Hinengaro is the superhero of our minds. She is our mind.

Hinengaro's name signals her mystery. Her gender is unmistakably female with the prefix 'Hine'. And while we always proceed with caution when looking at the components of kupu Māori, Māori words, it seems worthwhile here to consider the possible layers of meaning her name might reveal. The second aspect of her name, 'ngaro' carries resonances of being hidden, a sense of the undetected. The word 'whakangaro' means to put out of sight. Our phrase 'te wāhi ngaro', the hidden realm, the spiritual dimension, also helps us to understand how sacred the word 'ngaro' can be. It is hardly surprising that our source of thoughts and emotions, the wellspring of all ideas, dreams and aspirations, has a secluded and cryptic element.

Some of you might recognise the word hinengaro with a small 'h', often translated as the mind, awareness and consciousness. I have often wondered how Hinengaro lost her capital 'H'. Maybe it was deliberately taken away when translating Māori concepts into English and trying to find a close enough equivalent. You might know the word hinengaro from Te Whare Tapa Whā, the house with four walls, one of the most well-recognised metaphors used to explain our Māori ways of thinking about hauora, health and wellbeing. Commonly seen as a four-walled wharenui, a meeting house, the balance of all four sides represents the state of wellbeing we work towards. Te taha tinana is translated as physical health; te taha whānau stands for relationships; and te taha wairua emphasises our spiritual connection. These three structures stand alongside our taha hinengaro, representing the workings of the mind, to create this relatable framework.

And yet I have always felt that one of these things is not like the others. She is Hinengaro. Without Hinengaro, capital 'H', we cannot begin to understand the meaning of Te Whare Tapa Whā in the first place. Hinengaro is the one who enables us to imagine the whare and all of its parts, to make sense of the names and feelings and actions that flow from the four walls. Hinengaro leads us to question where this house has been built. On which whenua, on which land, with what history? Hinengaro is the one who gives us the words to express Te Whare Tapa Whā and hold that metaphor in mind, using it as a tool. She provides the myriad ways in which we experience our wellbeing.

Throughout my journey as a child and adolescent psychiatrist, I have tried to bring forward Hinengaro's gifts to serve our tāngata whaiora, our patients and whānau, offering all the learning that we discover together with Hinengaro as our guide. The lifelong journey of expanding medical and psychiatric skills is a constant companion. I also bring with me what I have been taught as a descendant of Muriwhenua and Ngāpuhi nui tonu, and as an ancestor of the future.

In 2008 I was privileged to be part of a wānanga in the Hokianga where we learned that one of the ways Hinengaro works is through 23 rua, or caves. Each cave has its own specific name, with uniquely tailored experiences invoking a different area of our minds which Hinengaro has chosen to prioritise. Her caves have a special, predetermined sequence. Hinengaro has made us this travel itinerary with a beginning, middle and an end; a departure gate, a series of essential places to visit, and a safe return. Hinengaro has designed her system of caves to be followed one after another, to take us deep down, to Te Whatumanawa, the bowels of the earth, within Papatūānuku, our earth mother, and back to the surface again. You might think of this as an ancient Māori underground pilgrimage. A subway or a metro system, where we get off at each stop to access her resources, to face her challenges and to be replenished.

We re-emerge from this mind journey with many insights into the heartbreak and sorrow, the pain and suffering of our lives.

In this way Hinengaro provides us with a pathway to gather her gifts and lessons, gaining further insights each time we choose to journey through these caves over the course of our lives. A uniquely Māori series of pre-arranged spaces where we can take our time to fully enter into new ways of thinking about thinking.

Why was I taught these resources? Over the years, I have deliberated about the responsibility placed in me. What is my part in ensuring this knowledge system is passed on in a useful and honouring way to serve others? How can I uphold the trust passed on by those who shared these precious taonga, these precious gifts? I have pondered how to bring this activity to life, how to write about the ways in which Hinengaro guides us to realise our potential in life through delving into her mind caves. How to ensure the legacy passed to me is available for future generations.

Since that wānanga in 2008, my imagination, one of Hinengaro's many superpowers, has been hard at work. I began to cautiously explore this interconnected system of caverns with tāngata whaiora, our patients, their whānau, and in my own life. Hinengaro has proven generous in opening up her treasures. This manaaki, this generosity, has continued to beckon, to invite visits into her caves. Such is her intent. Mind-gems gathered up to help us navigate our confusing and complex daily lives are there for a reason. She loves to host our visits. She loves to witness our growth, our shifting perspectives, our realisations.

Hinengaro gives us the extraordinary power to construct the caves as we go. She has been playing her own special version of Minecraft for a very, very long time. I imagine her renaming the game 'Min**d**craft'. I love the way Hinengaro uses her labyrinth of rua, carved deep in the earth, to remind us of our timeless connection with Papatūānuku, our earth mother. She draws us within Papatūānuku's bejewelled interior, to feel the fires of her fathomless, molten heart.

Hinengaro's gaze has allowed me to conjure up caves spiralling down, deep into Papatūānuku. Weaving around and around, and then curling back upwards until we return to the surface. Like running down a spiral staircase and back up again via a reverse twin spiral route. Each pathway with its own separate helical tunnel. Like a journey inside a pūpū harakeke, the flax snail precious to us in Te Tai Tokerau. This ancient takarangi, double-spiral journey, brings us deeper awareness, a renewed sense of clarity and purpose, and presses us to ask ourselves more useful, probing questions. Nourishing mind-food is Hinengaro's hākari, her feast. Just like kūmara pits that store our precious food, this ancient staple of life, passed down from our ancestors, made available whenever they are needed.

Have you ever been in a cave? For me, entering caves evokes a unique trepidation, a moving forward with caution. Leaving the world we are used to inhabiting, and entering a very different place. Caves are spaces that shut out the noise and the light we are used to. The distractions we rely on to drown out and numb our suffering are instantly removed. There is a feeling of raw exposure. Every breath seems so loud. Our senses heighten. We begin to notice aspects of our minds that have not been so readily available until now.

What has fascinated me over the years, drawing on the lessons in Hinengaro's rua, is that the creativity of the journey means we focus in unexpected ways on a broader range of opportunities and choices, on the widest expanse of possibility and potential in our lives. Hinengaro provides us with a spectrum of treasures in each of the interconnected caves. Hinengaro gives us the chance to recognise abundance and also the need to refuel. Some areas overflow with her riches. And sometimes Hinengaro's storage can become depleted. She helps us to see our natural strengths and to notice areas where our minds feel worn down. Hinengaro provides us with the mind-full sustenance we need throughout our lives. Delving into these caverns has opened up such an intense drive in me to create unique experiences that bring a visceral dimension to our mind-caving trip. A lived experience reflecting stories of our wheinga, our ancestors, and all of us as tangata whaiora, those who seek wellbeing.

Te Whatumanawa is the deepest place on our journey. The one place that is not strictly a cave. Te Whatumanawa signifies the concepts of both mind and heart. And it can mean the bowels of the earth. A flaming beacon of profound lessons in life, from the depths of Papatūānuku's molten centre. My father, John Elder, wrote a book called *The Bowels of the Earth* in 1976, published by Oxford University Press. Dad was a geophysicist. He was fascinated by the dynamics of rock formation over millennia, the way different layers and types of rock have danced, have collided and found their places alongside each other, for now. As I have delved into how to bring ngā rua o Hinengaro to life, my father has reminded me from beyond the arai, beyond the veil, that I have always loved ancient rocks, fossils and caves. I recognise Hinengaro's invitation into her places of wonder from my earliest memories.

~

Nau mai ki *Ara: A Māori guidebook of the mind.* A resource for our travels along this pathway into the bowels of Papatūānuku, the depths of Mother Earth, and back to the surface again. *Ara* is our navigational tool as we journey into ngā rua o Hinengaro, the caves of Hinengaro.

This book is my interpretation of Hinengaro and her 23 rua. A way to honour what was given to me and to hand this knowledge on in the hope that it can provide some comfort and ease in the chaos of our lives. Here are stories inspired by Hinengaro's superpowers from my work as a child and adolescent psychiatrist, as a mother and an aunty, as a daughter and cousin, as a descendant. Hinengaro has helped me to discover this ara, this path, bringing to life the wisdom of our tūpuna, our ancestors. Hinengaro's spiralling maze of rua takes us on new internal journeys. Learning about Hinengaro by traversing her rua opens up new possibilities, awakenings for all of us to uncover our own lessons. I hope this book provides you with a mind map that you can call your own.

Hinengaro, the Māori female deity of the mind, is here to help you to get to know your mind and to tell your own mind stories.

Nau mai, haere mai ki ngā rua o Hinengaro.

Welcome to *Ara*, your quest though the caves of Hinengaro.

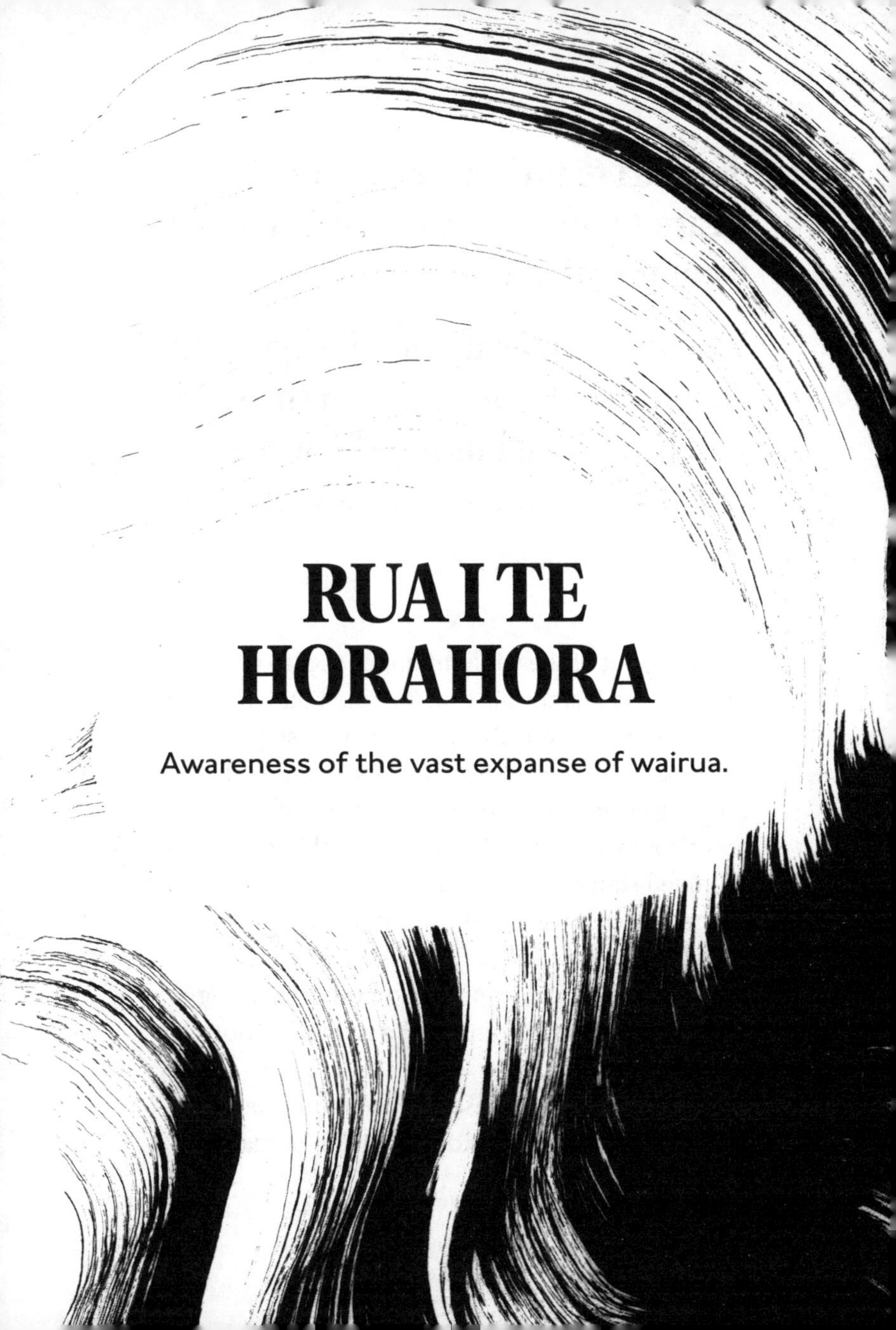

RUA I TE HORAHORA

Awareness of the vast expanse of wairua.

‘Ka pari te tai, ka timu te tai, ka ngaro te tohu i haea. Engari ka mau tonu te wairua.’

‘The tide comes in, the tide goes out, the line that was drawn in the sand will be hidden but not the wairua, not the lasting spiritual significance.’

— Pōroa, Te Rarawa kai whare.

Stepping out of the sunlight under the lip of this first rua, we feel the air cool on our skin. Hinengaro beckons us into a softly lit cavern. Our steps are a little tentative. Shells crunch under our feet. A growing curiosity builds as we sense that we are entering a vast network of caves. Looking up at the wrinkled skin of ancient rocks, there is an instant desire to touch the powdery and warm surface. This feels familiar. Like the reassuring touch of the palm of our kuia, our grandmother, holding us steady, we are heading in the right direction.

The welcoming incandescence surrounds us here, beckoning us deeper inside. We begin to make out sketches of spiralling forms. Drawings of intricate curving shells. Guides to their coiled internal worlds. Like maps of underground trains, they show the various stops where we disembark and explore. As our eyes adjust, we can make out the convergence of two steadily flowing streams gently glinting as they merge into the distance. Our wheinga, our tūpuna, have left us so many clues. This is how Hinengaro opens her first rua.

It feels apt to begin our journey with the famous whakatauākī, coined by Pōroa, one of our illustrious chiefs of former times. Pōroa's leadership continues to provide so much wisdom. So it is fitting that one of our ancestors from Te Hiku o te Ika, the tail of the fish, the Far North of Aotearoa, illuminates our experience, as we enter the first of Hinengaro's caves.

Pōroa made a decision, he drew a line in the sand. Despite the tides washing the line away, the wairua of the line he drew that day could never be erased and remains with us forever.

A battle was raging. Pōroa's wife, Whangatauatia, covered the dead body of her relation Te Kākā with her own to protect him from any further harm. Seeing her courage Pōroa abruptly ended the fighting, hence the words of his whakatauākī. His line in the sand would remain, despite being washed away with the tides. His resolution stands forever. To the north, lands were designated as Te Aupōuri, to the south Te Rarawa.

Rua i te horahora is the recognition that we come from wairua. Unlike the physical line in the sand, wairua can never be washed away. Wairua, the unique connection between people and the universe, some might say, our spiritual connectivity. We are wairua in physical form. Wairua people.

Wairua is where we always start. This focus on wairua awareness and knowledge returns us to the essence of ourselves, reminding us that wairua is critical to our wellbeing, to our view of the world and our place in it. To our perspectives about others. To our decisions and to our behaviour. To how we feel.

Here we breathe wairua.

It is no wonder Hinengaro starts us off with the wondrous sense of our wairua that transcends and transforms everything. Our innate sense of intuition and meaning.

We have arrived at a place filled with contemplation. A reminder that this is a place we can always visit, in less than a millisecond. Such is Hinengaro's speed and accuracy.

During my doctoral research in 2010, Dr Amster Reedy, a rangatira from Ngāti Porou, reminded me that we are a wairua people. Our spiritual lives are the basis of everything we do. Those wānanga, those discussions, taught me that wairua healing is the first thing that needs to happen for our whānau. Wairua healing is necessary to address the cultural injuries our wairua suffers. Cultural injuries demand a cultural response. The physical, psychological and relationship injuries all have a wairua component. Every aspect of loss of land and language, loss of knowing the names of our tūpuna, loss of Okoro and maramataka, the Māori lunar calendar — our way of experiencing time according to the natural world. Grief that we hide as we were taught to hate ourselves. Every rejection, every microaggression, every put-down and racist slur. Heaped up over generations.

People of all cultures carry their own spiritual burdens. Tyranny and war have created such intergenerational trauma around the world.

Hinengaro is leading us to the corners of her rua i te horahora, where collections of spiritual pain need to be processed and where the tools to begin healing reside.

Wairua is number one. Working with people suffering traumatic brain injuries and other forms of trauma means recognising whānau are also affected; these afflictions are experienced by all involved. I have learned that wairua is the tūāpapa, the basis, the foundation. The place from which we need to heal. Practices that strengthen our wairua are here in Hinengaro's rua i te horahora. Helping us to recognise any clutter we need to remove. Old wisdom carved in the strata of the rock face. The way forward marked out through the spiral-shell-staircases, left behind as loving ancestral clues on the walls of the cave. These are the gifts rua i te horahora offers.

Without Hinengaro we would not have the concepts with which we can express wairua. Hinengaro has given us the language, the letters to spell wairua's name. Hinengaro gives us the feelings that fan out before us here in this first cave of the journey. Hinengaro provides us with the tools and the space to process and find new splashes of meaning.

This is also the place where Hinengaro reminds us about death. The tiny creatures that once lived in the shells under our feet are long gone. Ngā wai e rua, the two streams flowing beside us, are our constant reminder of wairua. Wairua echoes in the ebb and flow of the tiny ripples on the rivulets' surface. In their watery murmurs we hear the sighs of wairua taking flight, the time when we pass away. Pōroa's whakatauākī speaks of death. The death of Te Kākā, and many others, forever part of that line in the wairua-sand of our memories.

So how can we use our time in rua i te horahora?

One way is to make sure we have kaumātua, our older people, in our thoughts, in our hearts, and if we are lucky, with us at the kitchen table, on our marae, in our late-night chats. Bringing their presence into our lives strengthens wairua.

Our Nanny, Annie Bowman née Yates, passed away when Mum was hapū, pregnant, with me. So I have got to know her through photos and stories. Her picture sits with her whanaunga, the photos of our beloved tūpuna, who watch over us at home. The stories of our old people who have passed on show us the many paths to realise the sources of our wairua strengths. Her hand holds mine in rua i te horahora.

Hinengaro reminds us that rua i te horahora has plenty of nooks and crannies where we can discover new ways to draw upon the experiences of our old people to help us with the challenges life throws our way. Our tūpuna continue to be on the journey with us. They invite us to join in weaving together the closeness of our whānau.

Do you know your grandmothers' stories? Or your grandfathers'? Or maybe it feels natural to start with aunts and uncles, or cousins. You might feel like starting with those close by, those who are still alive. Now is the time to begin to find out more about their lives. This is a practice that opens out Hinengaro's massive feast.

Maybe you can hear the old whispers, 'tohe roa, tohe roa', keep going, don't give up. Reach down to touch the ancient sands and precious shells, remembering Pōroa. The repetition of laughter-lines, the smiling curve of the toheroa shell, reminds us to retell these stories. Absorb the lessons from our grandparents. Take in the nourishment. The old people are waiting to pass on their powerful lessons to help us with daily life. Spend some time here. We can return again and again to our own tūpuna stories, finding more wairua insights, revealed in rua i te horahora. Who could be holding your hand while you explore the vast expanse of wairua?

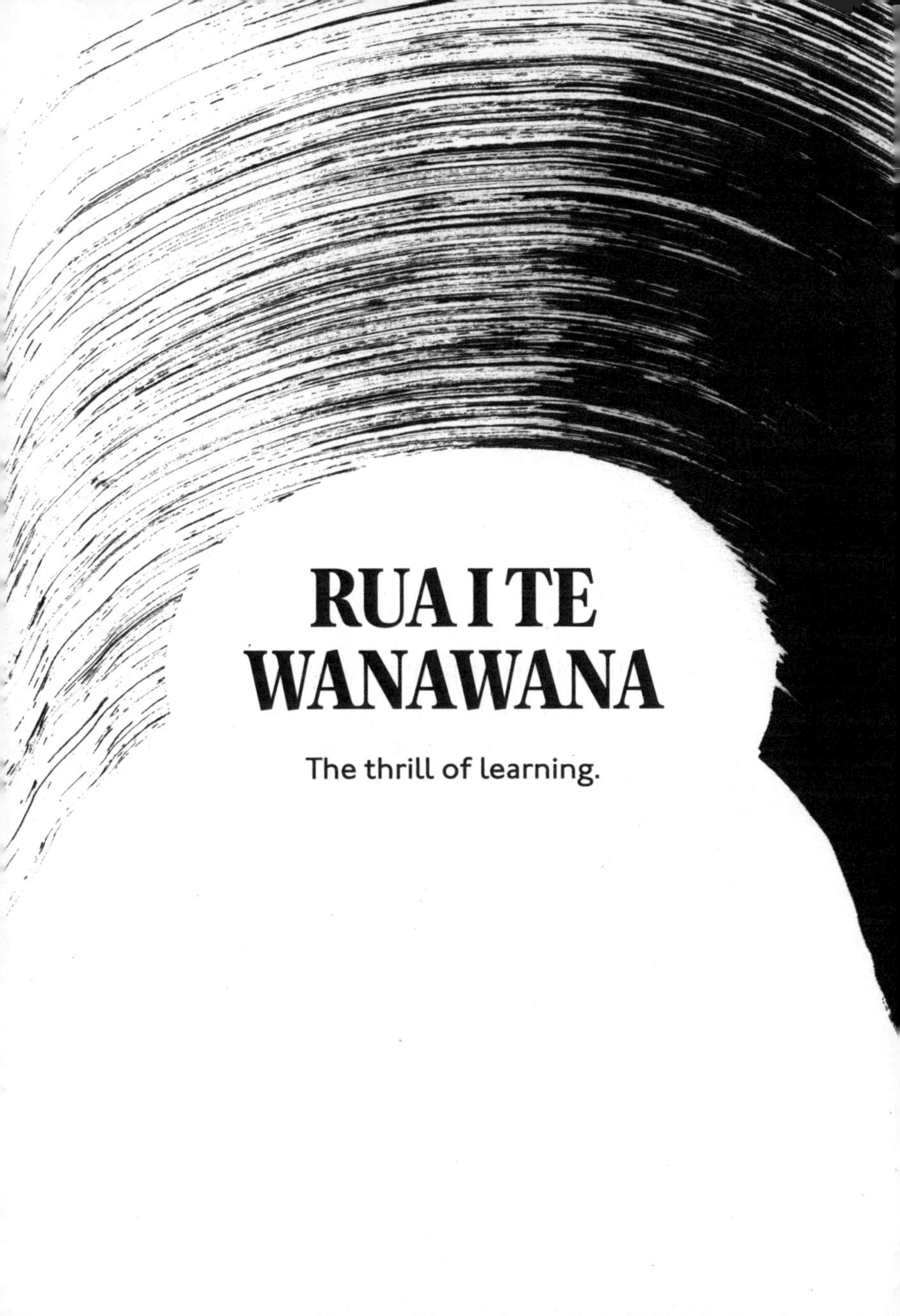

RUA I TE WANAWANA

The thrill of learning.

He ngākau hihiko te mokomoko.

The gecko is a creature fired up with excitement.

Following the sound of rippling water dancing through the time-honoured grooves in the rocks, our steps take us through a short tunnel. We can feel the vibration building, coming up through our feet. The ground is moving almost imperceptibly. A shuddering sensation all around, shaking us into a new sense of intense alertness and curiosity. The air is shimmering with excitement.

Tomo mai, ko tēnei te rua i te wanawana. Come in, this is rua i te wanawana.

Hinengaro envelops us in her formidable force-field. The energy surging through us is confronting. More proof that Hinengaro lives in our bodies too. We can feel our skin, our muscles, our puku and our hearts as her instrument, reverberating in awe. She awakens us into this quivering feeling of intoxication. Looking around we see glittering crystals on the cave walls. The beauty that surrounds us in this dazzling sanctuary. Irresistible questions are bubbling up from within, a bright curiosity that can't be denied. And we sense that we have company. Still not far from the surface, we have entered the home of the mokomoko, tiny geckos that dart in and out of the sequinned lights. Here under the gaze of a thousand reptilian eyes, we know we are being watched. Hinengaro has brought us into her thrilling hub of learning.

Learning is such a fundamental part of who we are. Here is a specific place to feel learning's pulse. Slightly unnerving at first, a strange intimacy. Hinengaro compels us to bring to the surface of our minds the myriad of learning possibilities that thrilling feelings ignite within us.

We all have this potential, this unique part of learning that we find completely absorbing and exhilarating. More than excitement, more than a happy contented sense of achievement. Pure fireworks pleasure.

Wanawana. It is a concept that is challenging to translate.

The repetition in the word itself is a valuable clue. The word 'wana' can indicate zeal, passion, verve, fervour. Doubling the word gives us a double dose of this pinnacle of fun-filled effervescence in things we love to learn.

Imagine if all learning was focused around this experience of wanawana. Imagine if the central question was: what learning excites you?

Recognising the kinds of learning that truly bring our wanawana essence to life opens up a completely different springboard from which to plunge, full-force, into our learning journeys. Our journey about what learning feels like.

Our mokomoko are Hinengaro's kaitiaki, guardians. They embody this exquisite thrill in learning. Mokomoko remind us that we have packed these truly excited moments away. Maybe we were taught early in our lives that learning was to be organised and controlled. There was no room, no time, for becoming passionate about certain subjects. No pathway to savour our own special thrilling moments in our learning. But here Hinengaro returns us to the awe we can feel when we learn something we love, something that fills us with purpose. Reminding us that the thrill we feel in learning is infectious. Once we experience those full-body waves of excitement in our learning, that same feeling spills out into other parts of our lives. This ultimate pleasure in learning fuels our hearts, propels our sense of direction. In this way we learn to love that experience of learning. To return to it again and again.

Remember how our tūpuna, would observe each mokopuna, each of their grandchildren and descendants. They paid close attention to what the babies and young children were drawn to. What do they revel in? Do they come alive in the depths of the ngahere, the forest, learning the names of different plants, the characteristics of the leaves, the various textures of tree bark, and their healing properties? Or are they most lively by the ocean, paying attention to the waves and currents? Or do they have an uncanny ability to recall where the stars rise and set? Do they prefer to listen and recount the stories of kaumātua, or are they quietly contemplative with an affinity for remembering karakia, prayers?

How do we reconnect with these feelings that we put aside when we were younger? Perhaps when we might have interpreted others' reactions as meaning they thought we were too full-on, and that we needed to tone ourselves down? Rua i te wanawana is a place for returning to times when we did not judge ourselves. When we were oblivious to the judgement of others.

How can we delve back into our memories of the awe-inspiring discovery of our fingers and toes? The fascination and joy we experienced. Perhaps long forgotten, then reignited when we see our tamariki mokopuna and experience their delight and fascination at their discoveries. The life lessons of crawling and walking, running, jumping on a trampoline, learning to speak and sing, to cartwheel and roll, to pūkana and swim, to read and write, to imagine other worlds. With the reclaiming of our thrill in early experiences of learning, mistakes and all, we begin to sense the incredible lessons that are stored here in this rua. We have learned so much, witnessing the thrill of learning in others and we can now feel these unique gifts absorbed so deeply within ourselves. These are the riches that rua i te wanawana brings into our lives.

For me, exploring the stories from our own people provides this unquenchable rua i te wanawana effect. Pausing here, we sense our part in the intricately woven meanings. We can reach out and grip onto their inviting trailing threads, following their lead into the richly woven whāriki, those lovingly threaded mats. Feeling our own life adventures stitched in with their intergenerational tapestries of stories. Discovering their lessons for us, here in today's world.

One of those threads for me has been learning about Te Kākā, one of our Te Aupōuri chiefs, and how he kept his mokomoko, his geckos, as pets. These descriptions take me on a vivid learning adventure. These creatures were highly sensitive to movement. At the slightest vibration, their reactions would alert Te Kākā to possible threat from unwelcome visitors. Tū te wanawana is also the name for the atua of reptiles, the deity that rules these creatures. This aspect of wanawana helps us to remember the power of these ancient beings — their so-called 'parietal eye', their third eye, unique in sensing the light and darkness, in this world and beyond. A sudden flash of movement at the edge of the cave draws your attention. Out of the corner of your eye, the quivering tail of a tiny lizard disappears into the shadows. A surge of adrenaline. An unexpected shiver of excitement.

Hinengaro reminds us that learning has a unique thrill that is such a potent force in our lives. We are all capable of being awe-struck. This propels us forward, gives us hope and energy and fuels our resourcefulness.

Hinengaro invites us to reconnect with our own unique wanawana, our own thrilling feelings, when we learn something that truly excites us. To remember our rare abilities when we learn what makes us feel most alive. To be brave and explore strengthening our own language and cultural practices, te reo Māori me ōna tikanga; to learn mahinga kai, gardening and providing fresh vegetables for the whānau. Learning waiata, haka, mōteatea. Getting back into the sports you loved at school, even though the knees might be a bit older now, maybe as a coach or an umpire? Perhaps some aspect of art or music, weaving, or singing, composing songs for your mokopuna yet to be born? What do you want to learn more about that really whets your appetite? Have you been reminded of something you loved to learn, but put away because you felt you didn't have time for that anymore? How could you harness the thrill of learning in your everyday life, like the flicking tail of your very own mokomoko?

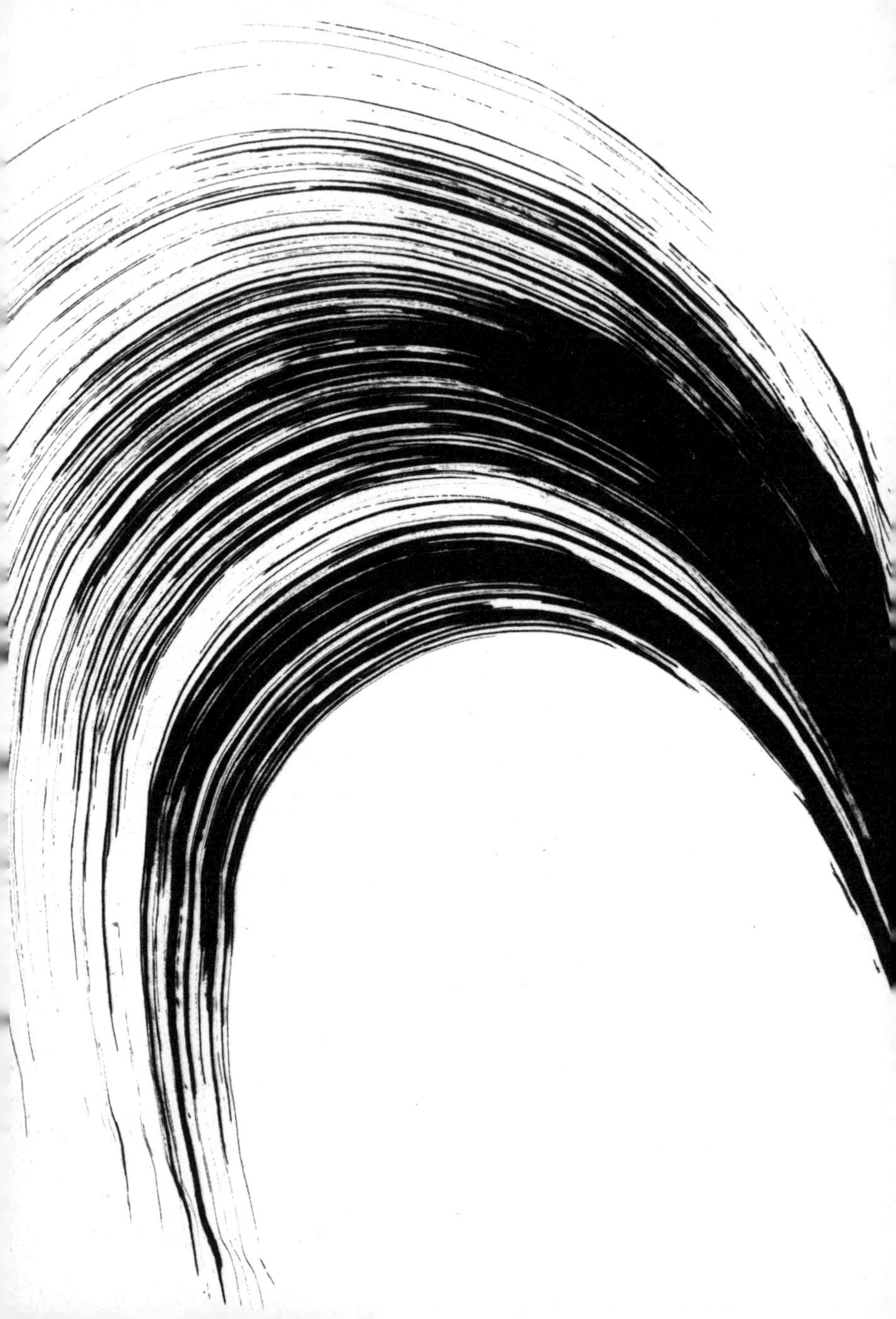

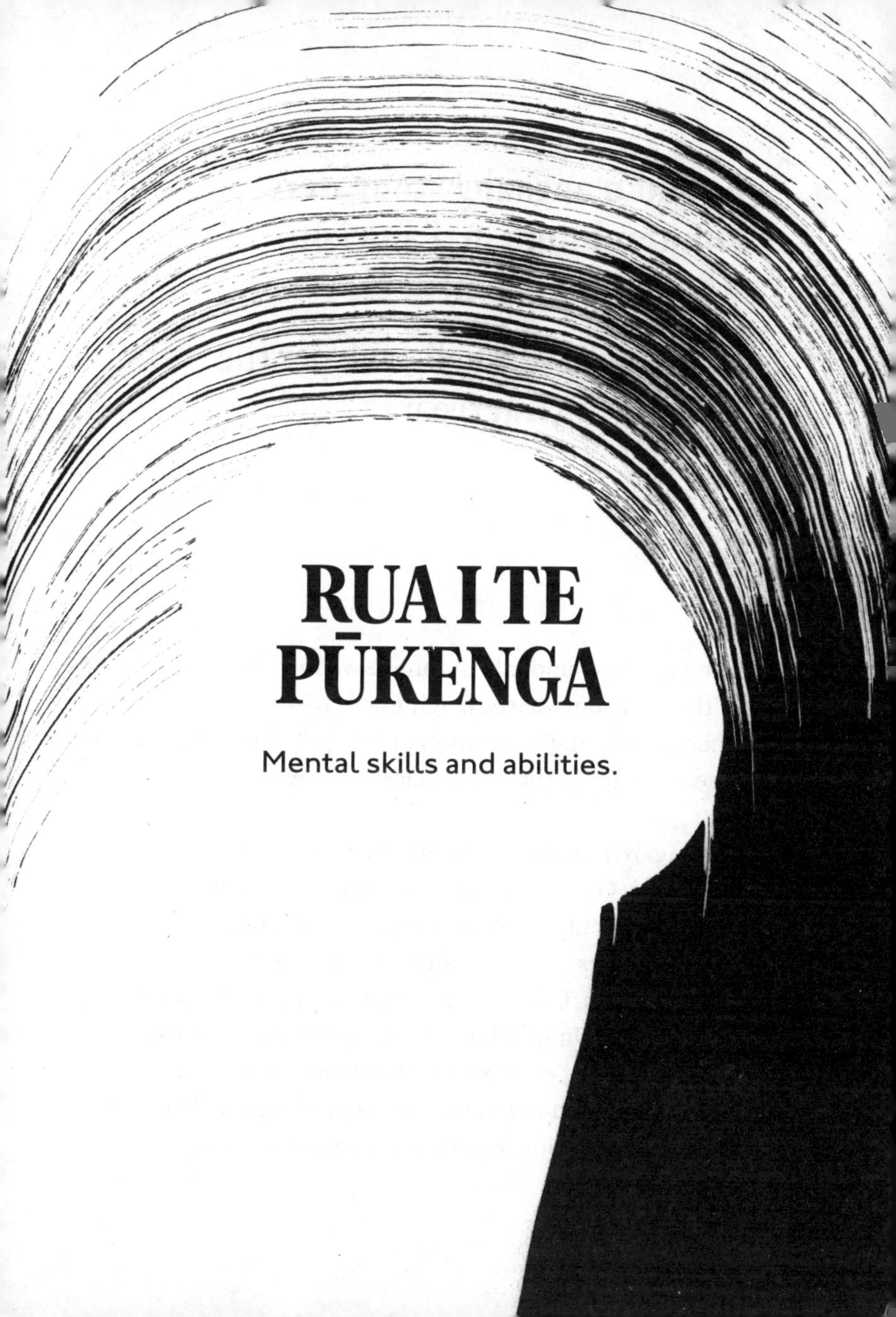

RUA I TE PŪKENGA

Mental skills and abilities.

Kei taku angaanga tongarerewa, kōhumuhumu mai ana i ōu whakaaro nui o neherā.

My beloved seashell, whisper the wisdom of yesteryear.

The light has suddenly dimmed. We inch forward in the dark, our senses heightened. Disorientated. There is a strange sensation of not quite knowing where we are in time and space.

Hinengaro envelops us in another mysterious challenge. Our breathing quickens. Our hearts are beating out a deafening drum solo in our ears. Our eyes strain to catch any clues as to our surroundings. Our fingers stretch out in desperation to the walls. Undulations of seashells meet us. How strange and yet comforting. Remnants of ancient feasts layered in the rock. The signs of sharing kai, abundance, the joy of working together, passing on what we know, strengthening our bonds. Our fear is replaced. We are not alone. Through the touch of skin on shell, our fingertips read the ocean's braille of togetherness. These clues transport us across time; past, present and future all at once.

Hinengaro uses the darkness and unfamiliarity of rua i te pūkenga, the trepidation of uncertainty, as we enter, forcing us to hone our focus, to highlight that we have skills and that our skills are amplified when we work as one. Here, our recognition of the shells from these so-called kitchen middens, these powerful reminders, transport us to places and times where we can feel all of our mental proficiency come to life. Our fingerprint scans open the barnacle-encrusted lid to a box of tools. A chest filled with a whole system of mental skills ready for us to practise.

Hinengaro awakens ancient memories. In an instant she transports us, and we are standing barefoot on timber slabs, astride a waka hourua, a double-hulled waka, the rhythm of the rolling waves somehow comforting. We can see, far away in the distance, some puffy white clouds hovering above a tiny speck of land. A familiarity rises in our chests. We have always known that land is there, waiting for us to hoist those maunga, those mountains, up out of the sea. Droplets of sea spray whip against our cheeks, the salt catching in our lashes; we feel our hands gripping tight as we pull the land closer towards us. We are not alone. Our whānau are here on the waka with us. Some we recognise only from photos. Some we have never seen before. And yet the momo, the old traits, tell us we are blood. Smiling faces as we work together to fish up the whenua which grows closer and closer, higher and higher over the horizon. This whenua that we have practised drawing towards us in our dreams.

Without realising it, we have closed our eyes and as we open them, we find the light is growing in the cave. The seashells layering the walls are clear now. Pearly in places, flecks of pāua flickering with iridescence. The cave feels like one massive shell curving with its single ear, tuned to a faint murmuring tide, only just audible.

This is the place where Hinengaro reminds us of our many mental skills and abilities. She likes to make it clear that this is a whole-of-body experience. We feel her domain extending throughout every pore, every cell in our bodies and beyond.

Hinengaro always starts us off in the dark here. Forcing us to create a myriad of scenarios so we can begin to assess any situation, any challenge. She starts us from scratch. There is so much freedom for us to move our thoughts and feelings around unfettered. Even when we are scared, and we might want to run and hide, she holds us in this place. Hinengaro reminds us that we have the know-how, we will work it out. And she can bring a pause in the urgency. There can be a moment of peace at any time, no matter the raging storms of our lives. Tempests that rush though our bodies, making purposeful thoughts feel out of reach. We can still see what is happening from different points of view. Like the curvature of the shells, the emerging light refracting in different patterns, there are many points to focus on. So many places where we can find solutions. And we know our ability to grow ingenuity has a collective heart. Joined up, forever connected. Here we are filled with reminders that the skills of our forebears are available. Hinengaro brings their attributes into our embrace.

Hinengaro provided our vivid waka experience to reinforce what is right here in rua i te pūkenga. The multiple ways we can bring forward exactly what we need from the experiences of old. Just like being on the ocean and recognising the signs of land in the distance, and using these navigational tools to surge ahead, to meet our destination. We know we need to do much more than set goals. We remember the frustration when our goals were too easy to reach, when we set our own expectations too low. And the humiliation we feel when we don't reach the goals we planned. Hinengaro reveals the wealth of our sheer power and brilliance, our shared mental mastery. Hinengaro is magnificent. These are the generous gifts in our shell-encrusted rua i te pūkenga.

Take a moment to think of a seashell, a descendant of Tangaroa, deity of the ocean. Maybe you have a favourite treasure you can hold in the warmth of your hand? You can feel all the ancient layers of skill, the minute particles assembled with such precision. Notice its tiny details as a metaphor for the incredible mastery you too can build on. Expressions of all of those who you can work with to expand and hone your own craft. Starting from a place of darkness and fear, you now have reminders of a system of abilities, just as the small sea creature crafted its beautiful home from minuscule elements of the sea. No matter how much anxiety you feel, you have such a wide range of possibilities to consider and share with others. Pausing, breathing, allowing this collective approach for expertise to begin to take shape. Just like the crafting of such a seemingly simple yet elegant house for a tiny offspring of Tangaroa. Seashells will always be your talisman, connecting you to your very own system of pūkenga. A reminder of the abundance of abilities Hinengaro has ready for you. Right at your fingertips.

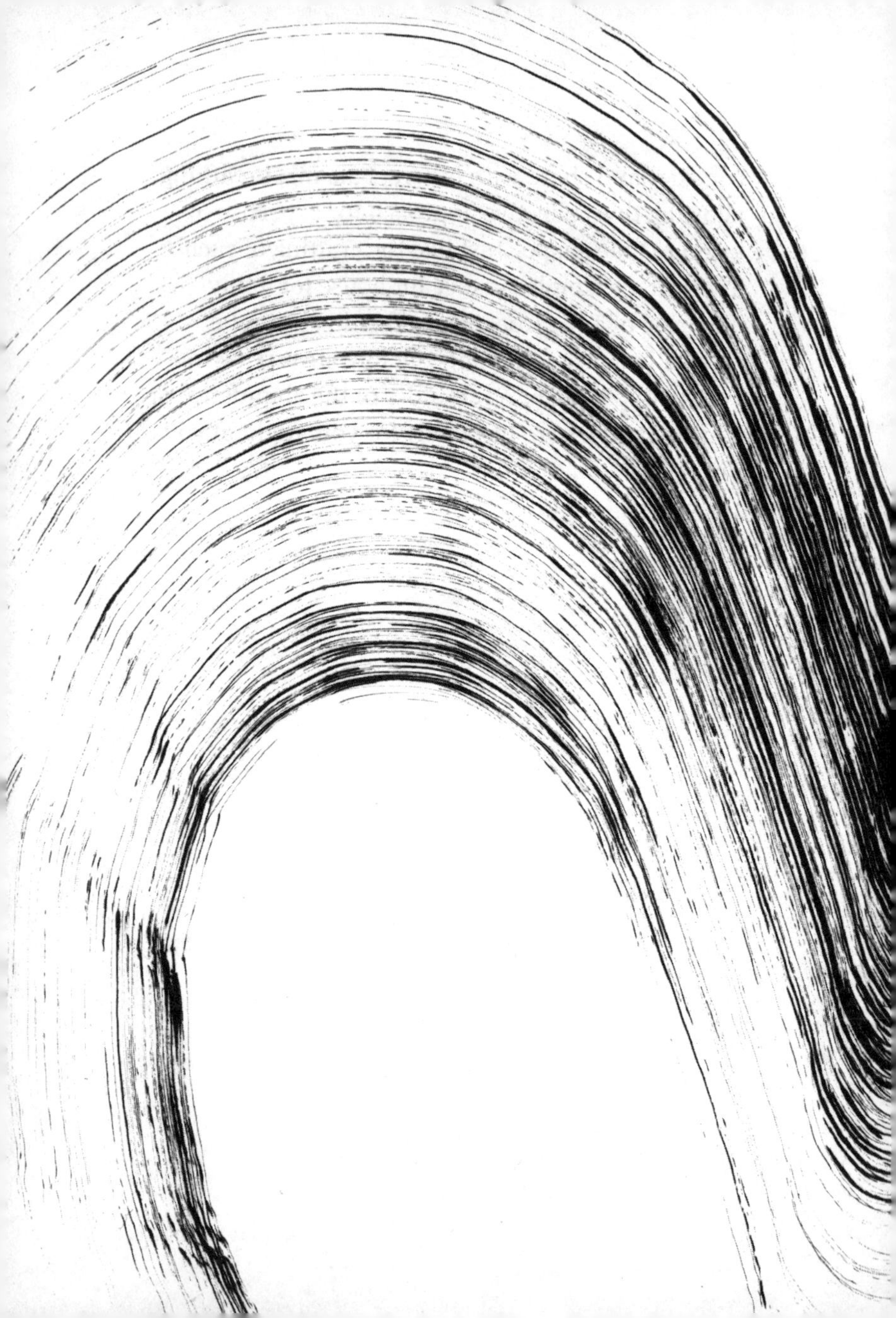

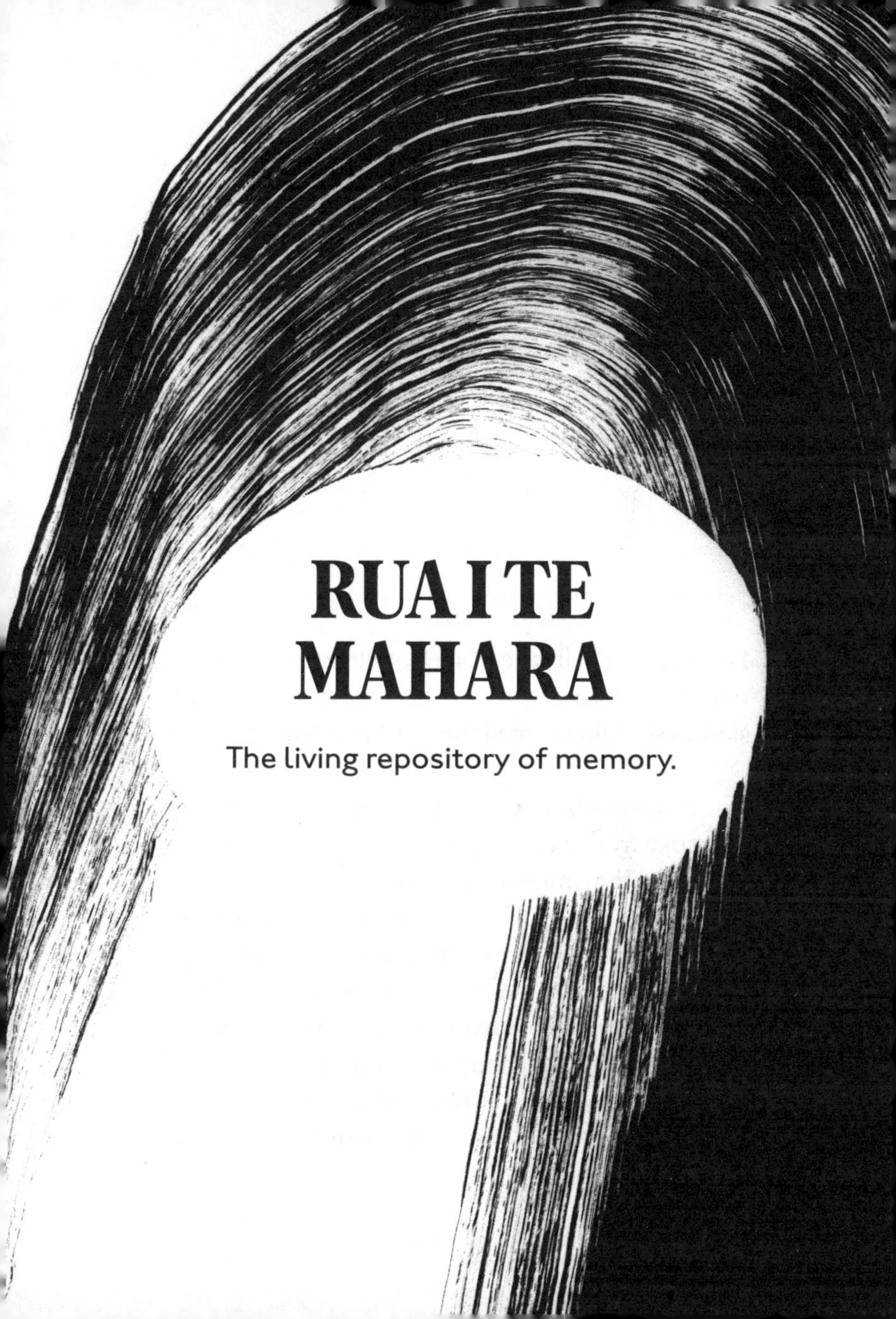

RUA I TE MAHARA

The living repository of memory.

He kitenga kanohi, he hokinga mahara.

A face from the past brings back emotion.

Leaving our shell cave, rua i te pūkenga, feeling a refreshed sense of working together to improve our skills, we begin to smell the most beautiful fragrance.

Our noses are tickled with the merest suggestion of smoke from a cooking fire. Or is it? No wait, of course, the unmistakable waft of hāngī steam. Instantly the memories flood in, just as the saliva threatens to flood our mouths. Pictures cascading through time, like old-fashioned movie reels. Grins and belly-laugh tears from all those hāngī prep moments. Peeling, chopping, sorting out portions, all the while cackling at the stories from our aunties, our nannies, our cousins and uncles. Their faces ride back into memory on our eager taste buds, longing for just one more perfect, buttery mouthful of our younger days.

The unexpected tendrils of our favourite cooking smells welcome us into the rua i te mahara. The storehouse of memory. A place of such surprises. Dappled light creates movement in the crevices of the rock walls, shifting our focus, demanding our attention and fuelling our curiosity. This is a cave of mirror-like shimmer, sudden points of light contrast with unpredictable shadows. Gleaming reflections target our memories as they wax and wane. Recollections from different angles play in the light for a while, only to dissolve into obscurity. Some recollections are clear and persistent, while others are only momentary, a fleeting glimpse in our peripheral vision.

Memory is our superpower. Our old people could recall and recite whakapapa, genealogy, for days. They had incantations that lasted all night. Hinengaro reminds us that we can come back here at any time to stand in the boundless, dancing light of memory. Here we reclaim our memory strengths. On one hand we witness remembrance with such vitality, bouncing from one reflective surface to another, recapturing so many moments of time gone by, alongside what happened milliseconds before. On the other, we also feel the pull of memory's escape out of sight. The refracting play of light and shadow somehow strengthens our recognition, our beliefs and our awareness of how important it is to take care of memory. To take care of the gifts from rua i te mahara.

Some memories fade, and this is a blessing. The famous saying, 'he taonga te wareware', 'to forget is a gift', is reflected back in one looking-glass. A sigh of gratitude for the fading memories of some of our life experiences. The relief we feel that we can't remember the totality of pain in childbirth. Just as well, or we might only ever have one child.

Other kinds of pain and suffering carry different kinds of memories, becoming lodged in fractured, splintered-off fragments, which Hinengaro could not yet completely obscure. Some must come into the light first before they can drift away into the wings of life's stage. These memories can emerge unexpectedly and cause us so much distress.
We pass through ngā rua i horahora, wanawana, pūkenga, to best prepare us for the respect we must have for the power of memory.

Activating our memory has rules. Breaking karakia, breaking the recitation of lines of whakapapa was forbidden. There were dire consequences for such infractions. Such was the utmost importance given to the memory of the correct order of these esoteric and sacred elements of knowledge. As for those recalling the recipe for fry bread, some might see this as more mundane but nevertheless, it is crucial. Get it wrong and you know there will be hell to pay.

Here in this cave of magic we revolve as the light and shade leaps from surface to surface. We become part of the orbit of our Okoro, our maramataka, the cycles of our moon. Seeing our lives through the eyes of Hina, our moon goddess. We are standing at the centre of a stage. A central turntable slowly revolves. Hinengaro reminds us with each revolution that we are ageing, and as we age memories can begin to slip into the shade. The actions we have relived so many times from the past might be spared. Often it is the new memories that are first to fade.

Under which of Hina's faces were you born? It is fascinating to find out and then to begin to collect memories from that moon phase with every passing month. In that way we call to mind our growth, weaving memories of life's orbiting cycles. I was born under a Huna moon. For me, our Huna moon harks back to that first breath. 'Me aro koe ki te hā o Hineahuone', 'pay heed to the dignity of women'. This marks the first expansion of the lungs. The Huna moment, where the magic of life happened. Readiness in the pause before planting, the moment of suspension before putting our plans into action.

We collect memories every year when we celebrate our own birthdays on a different moonday from when Hina's face first greeted us. It struck me that we only celebrate our birth-moon every 30 years. I didn't get to celebrate my birthday-moon on Huna again until I was 30. And I look forward to seeing Huna again on my birthday when I am 60. Quite a different way to ruminate on the memories over such great intervals of our lives. Some of us might celebrate two such birthdays and maybe a few might see three. What memories do you most cherish, perhaps thinking about when in the lunar calendar they occurred? Do you worry your memories will be lost with your passing? How could you keep them alive? What are the cooking smells, the fragrances of your youth? How could you share these recollections and reflections, these mirrors into the world of your life with your whānau? Tell your stories, write them down, record them for your mokopuna. Create opportunities to keep memory in mind.

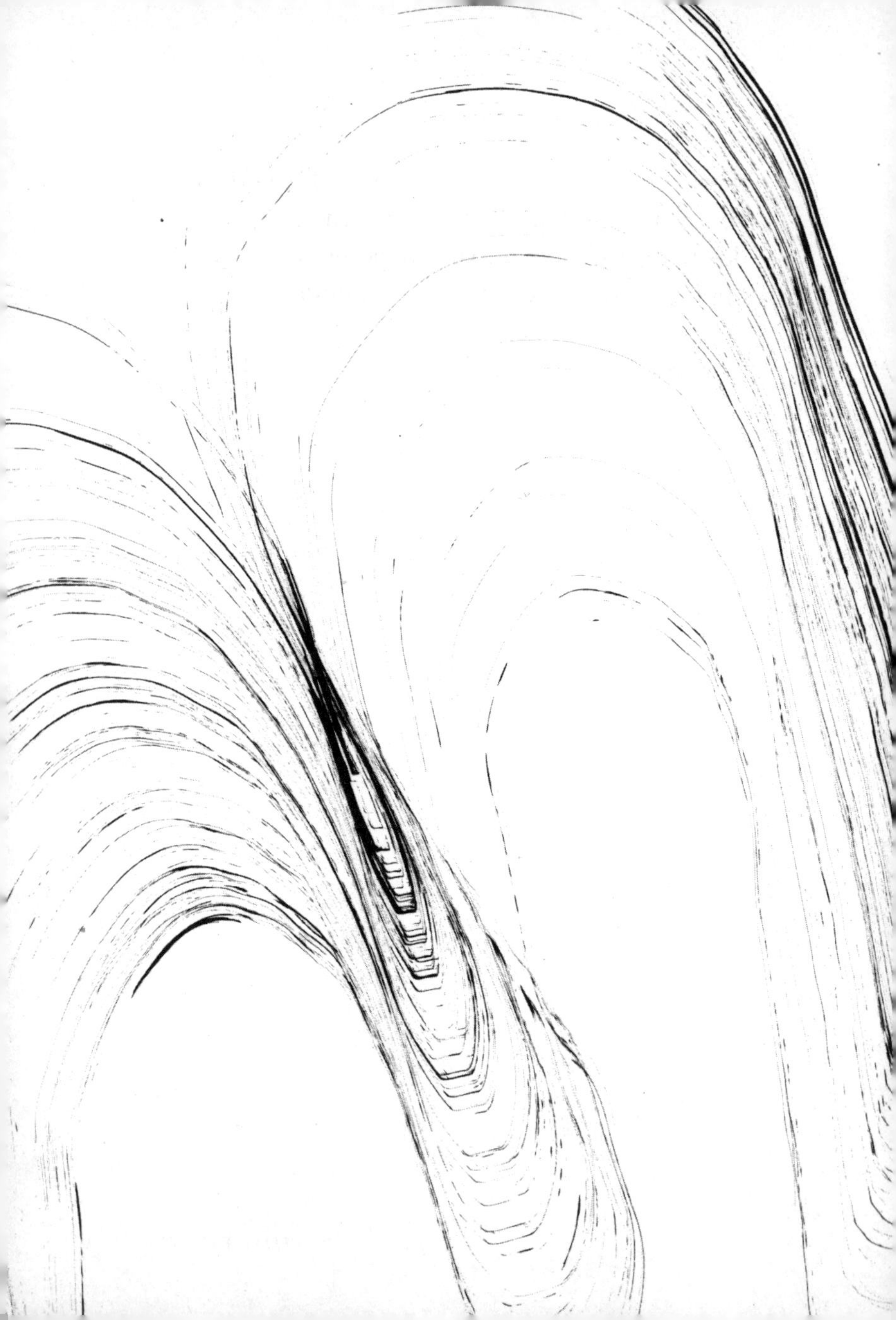

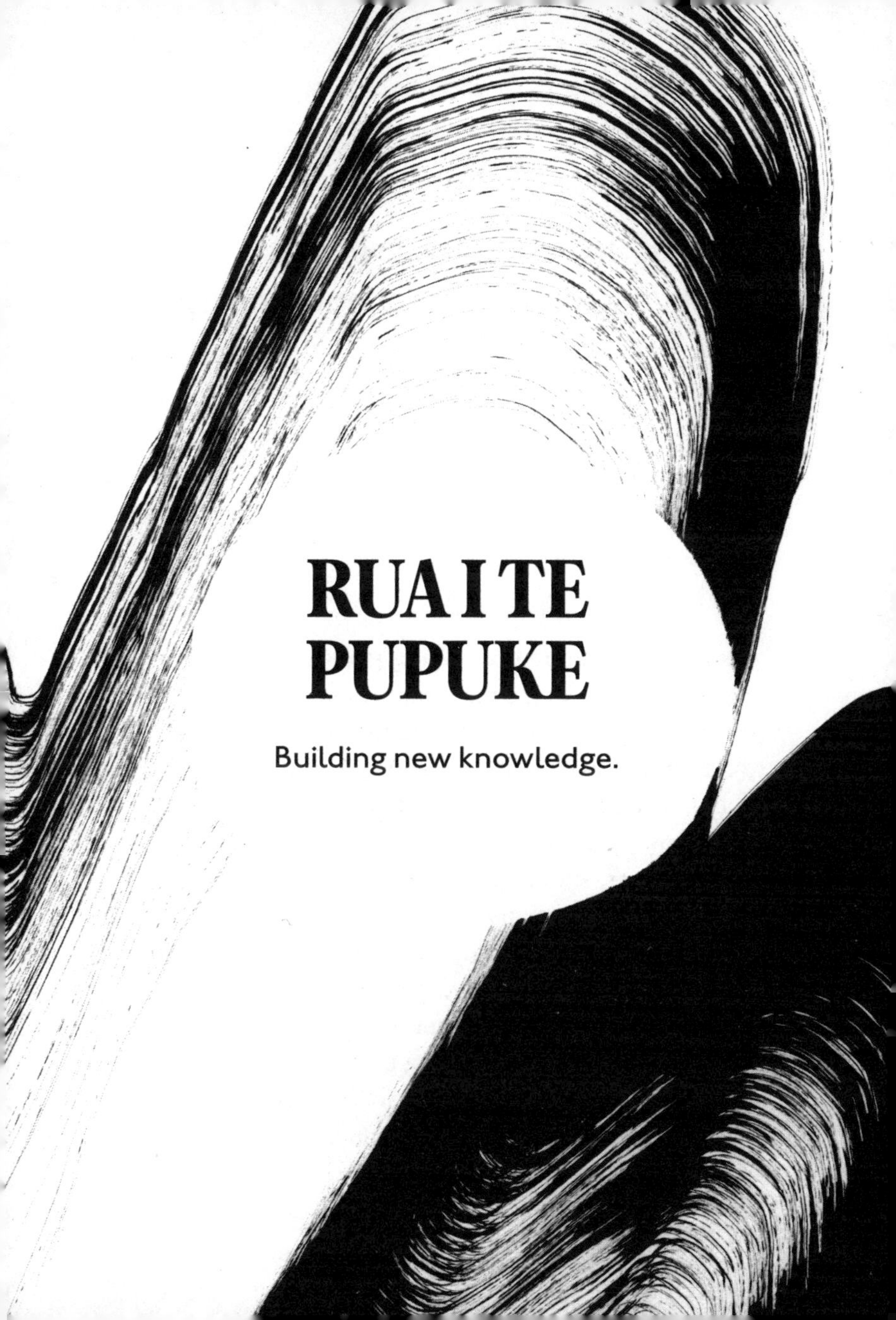
RUA I TE
PUPUKE
Building new knowledge.

Ko Tāne te Pupuke.

An exciting abundance of new thoughts and plans are building up.

As we leave behind the looking-glass alchemy of memory in rua i te mahara, majestic rock formations suddenly rise from the darkness. At first, they resemble huge shadowy figures. We halt abruptly. Hinengaro demands our courage. The growing golden light reveals these are in fact stone pillars, standing proudly in the light of a thousand glow-worms. Monumental columns of rock pushing their way upwards. Stalagmites rising like enormous waxy birthday candles. Waves of stone droplets seem to linger as they drip down their sides, the pou stretching ever higher. In the distance we see what look like whānau groups of these stone-tree formations. Some freshly made, just starting out, heaped up in tiny hillocks, yet to find their true stature. Others, more developed, filled with promise. In some places, these great rocky efforts are greeted by their relations, the stalactites. Stony icicles, hanging from the vaulted ceiling, as if a frosty blast had suddenly suspended the flow of water from the cave's ceiling way above our heads. In some places the edges of their rocky fingernails touch each other like acrobats' hands, finding each other in the silence.

We have entered rua i te pupuke. Hinengaro has dedicated this special place to storing all of her tools to build new learning and to embrace the welling up of emotion that arises from the experience.

We see new learning depicted for us in these strangely beautiful stone statues. They remind us there is a powerful reciprocity that comes from all around us and from within ourselves when we are building new thinking. Hinengaro shows us these alternative points of view in her own special way. Her rocks lead by example. They show us how to take time, moving at a slow, deliberate pace. Their calm presence slows our breath, their influence compelling. We need the longer-term view to build our knowledge layer by layer. A view that spans generations. The stones are not perfectly formed in their growth either. Just like us, they have their glorious imperfections. Rocky growth patterns that seem to veer off in a different direction for a while. There is exploration. No matter where they started from, there is a never-ending persistence of movement into the void. Growth is not a straight line.

Stalagmites rise up from the floor, stand in their perspective, hold their position, and forever build upwards from their initial premise. Their opposites, stalactites, are suspended chandeliers in stone, responding according to the force of gravity. Somehow there is a growing together of views. I imagine each reaching towards the other in their vehemently held ideas. Holding to their own vision. And after a thousand years of debate and argument, sometimes they meet, sometimes they keep their distance.

I wonder how these rock formations communicate. How are they responding to each other's growth? How do they know they have the chance to meet in the middle of the vast space of this rua i te pupuke?

Our own challenging, inspirational and, at times, disturbing ideas may be a response to provocative ideas from others. Perhaps this new learning is unexpected, we might feel forced to learn new things, under pressure, under unforeseen conditions. Maybe on the surface a new way of looking at things could be disguised as something rather routine. First glance might suggest this is a bit tedious, perhaps. But we sense all is not as it seems. New learning is triggered by both dramatic events and those that seem simple enough, at least to begin with. New learning demands our attention. After a while we start to realise we must activate learning to find out more about what is making us toss and turn at night, to discover more about what creates disturbance in our lives.

Emotions about this kind of challenge to our thinking are sometimes frowned upon. But why shouldn't we care deeply about the things that matter the most and about the new learning that we are propelled to undertake? Why the pressure to behave as if we don't care about our learning, that this doesn't really matter? Priorities are held with passion, especially when they are threatened or disregarded. Escalation of new ideas is infused with emotion. The occasional breakthrough of 'aha' moments. The shedding of the old thinking, past its use-by date. Often, we find that disappointment and irritation, the fear of making mistakes, the rush to latch onto the first workable solution, and then the fear to admit we were wrong kicks in. The churn in our puku, our stomachs, when we come so close to success. Hinengaro is across all of this, mind and body.

Quietly absorbing the needs of new learning and the rush of emotions we feel here, standing in Hinengaro's rua i te pupuke encourages us to remember the elements from the previous caves we have been through. The intensity building in layers of insight.

Rua i te horahora, the invisible wairua filaments that fan out all around us, linking us to the entire universe; rua i te wanawana, the thrill of learning; rua i te pūkenga, our mental skills; rua i te mahara, the importance of memory: these rua have each provided their gifts to set us up for how we experience rua i te pupuke.

This is a place to consider what we have been taught about how the mind works. To investigate ideas of the mind from our own cultural backgrounds. A place to recognise that we are all capable of getting stuck in a particular mindset. To consider how we could use imagination and creativity to shift the stickiness of our minds.

Hinengaro asks us to examine the range of pressures we face which expose the need for unlocking our pre-existing limitations of thinking, what we have done in the past and what we could think about differently next time.

She reminds us that emotions are not a weakness. Our feelings show we care. Our affections are a useful yardstick — they reveal how to build our new knowledge with heart.

Maybe you haven't thought about rocks moving and changing shape before. Maybe you have just noticed new ideas and new feelings emerging from your experiences here in rua i te pupuke. This is Hinengaro's invitation to make a regular time to grow your new thoughts about how you think and feel. You might be someone who likes to jot these down, or to record them as voice notes. You might like to draw or paint your own interpretation of rua i te pupuke. Maybe share it with those around you, with your whānau perhaps, as a way to promote discussion and add more layers of new learning and the feelings you are unlocking.

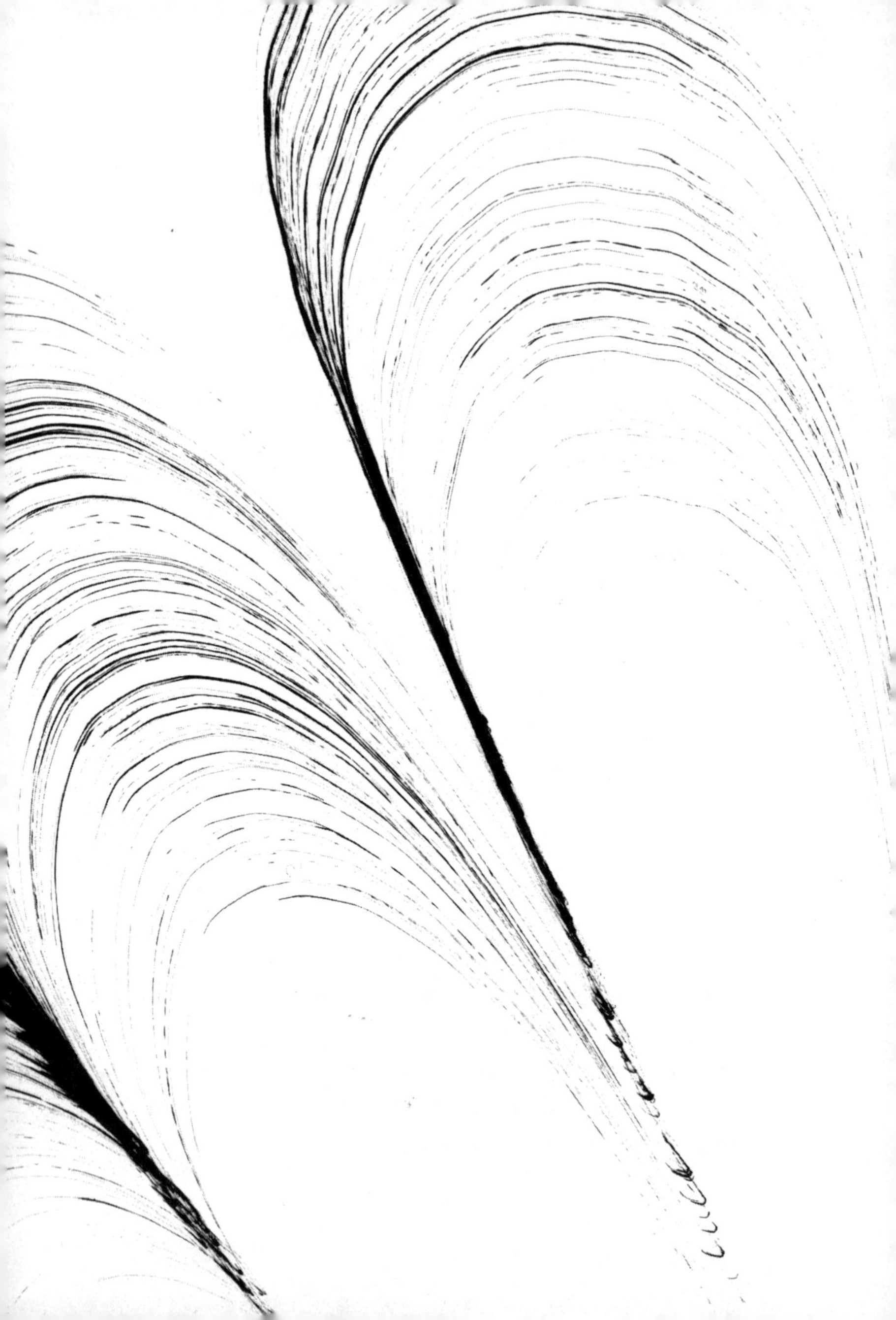

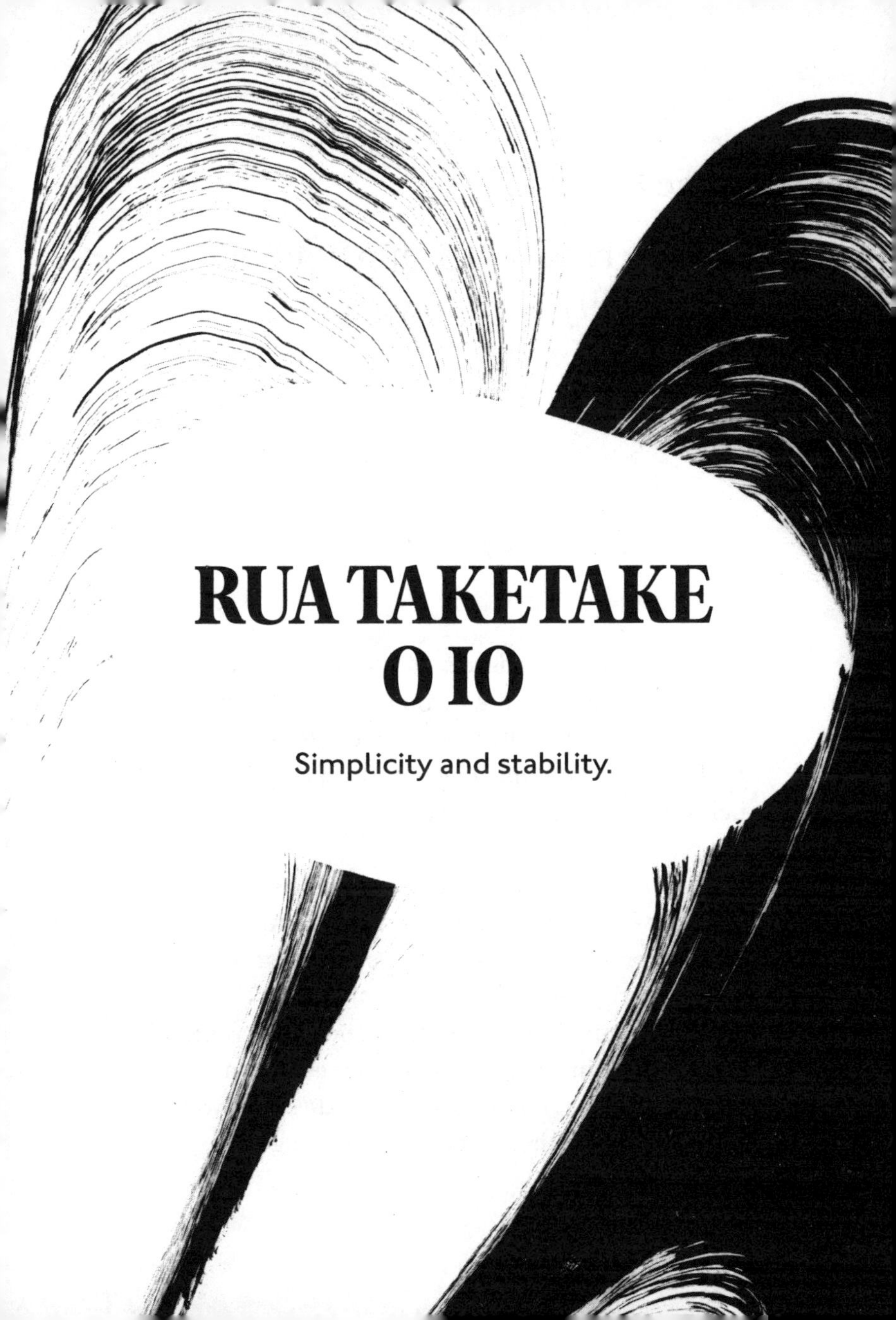

RUA TAKETAKE O IO

Simplicity and stability.

Me he tao waka.

Like the ballast of a ship, finding the stability of our own waka.

A wave of solemnity descends. Pausing at the entrance, we absorb the further slowing of time. Smooth obsidian walls meet our hands as we carefully step into this new rua, the glassy black rock somehow deeply reassuring.

We have become more accustomed to the caves now. Our eyes have matured in their ability to see into the shadows. Here we become aware of a natural clarity beyond the sense of vision. There is an air of balance. A quiet sense of peace surrounds us. A contrasting spark of light pierces the dark from high above. Filaments of delicate spiderwebs shimmer in the ethereal beam. Following the light's direction, we find a place to sit. It is as if we are pulled down into the rock, our bones sinking into the huge stone sofa. A gentle ease descends. Life's complications fall away. The boulder's curves hold us within their spacious arms. How can a rock feel soft? Our whole weight — emotional, physical, spiritual weight — is absorbed. This place lets it all sink in. The fullness, the stretching of the space we occupy in the world comes to rest here.

Io, sometimes referred to as Io matua kore, the being with no parents. The beginning. The source of creation. In some parts of Te Tai Tokerau, this is how we describe the origin of everything. Io for short. Hinengaro has prepared this rua so that we can begin to experience our kinship with Io. Io brings the weight of realisation, that we are a minuscule link in the long whakapapa nets of connection. Io reminds us of this infinite perspective. We feel the strength in being so small in the greater scheme of things. Our place in the order of things is simple and straightforward. There is an acceptance of the permanence of whakapapa, and this acceptance brings a freeing of possibility to navigate our stress and fear with integrity.

Feeling our direct line of connection to Io replenishes us with generations of attempts to be open and to face fears about taking responsibility for decisions. Our ability to follow through on what we said we would do. Here is the source of our stability in learning from admitting our mistakes.

Rua taketake o Io feels like a tao waka; the cave of the ancient one has the characteristics of the ballast of a ship. Simplicity and stability. The serenity of a place dedicated to the very beginning. We feel the dignity of the place, he pēhanga kōhatu, the ballast of rocks, the weight of stability.

Where do we find that sense of this ballast, holding our own waka on track when we might feel like we are being buffeted around in the sea of life? How can we identify the stories that provide equilibrium with which we can build unity and cohesion? We come to this rua better prepared than we might think at first. We have shut out the noise of the world, just for a while. We have experienced a new way to draw on the abundance that Hinengaro's rua have brought to our attention. Deliberately letting simplicity be our guide is another defining act to let our experiences of life settle into place.

One of the stories of simplicity that I find inspiring is part of Tūmatahina's legacy. He is well known for using the example of kuaka, godwits, to help our people see how to work together to reach safety. Our old people paid attention to these birds, who were known for their long migrations across the world and back again to Muriwhenua, our shared home in the far, Far North. Our ancestors revered the birds' attributes of persistence and working together. These continue to be seen as human traits uniquely available to our people and worthy of emulating. Another one of Tūmatahina's clever strategies was to ask the others to step into his massive footprints to make it look as though only one person was getting away. I often think about how we can leave footprints for others to follow, so there can be a natural, easy progression in the development of ideas and whānau wellbeing. A potent way to imagine what we leave behind for our descendants. Where do our footsteps end so others can take the journey from here?

We follow in the footsteps of Io.

Here in Hinengaro's rua taketake o Io we can begin to pay attention to the whakapapa footsteps Io has left for us. That long journey from the origin of whakapapa which we all add to along the long beach of life, death and beyond.

How can you identify a sense of gravitas, the moments of poise where you can find your own equilibrium? Where do you find your emotional gravity? This question might lead you to set up some regular whānau hui, extended-family meetings, or meetings with friends to find language for the ways to form this deep experience of feeling grounded. This rua provides such deep reassurance, a place from which to reaffirm the ways you want to talk about the serious concerns in your life and what to then do about them.

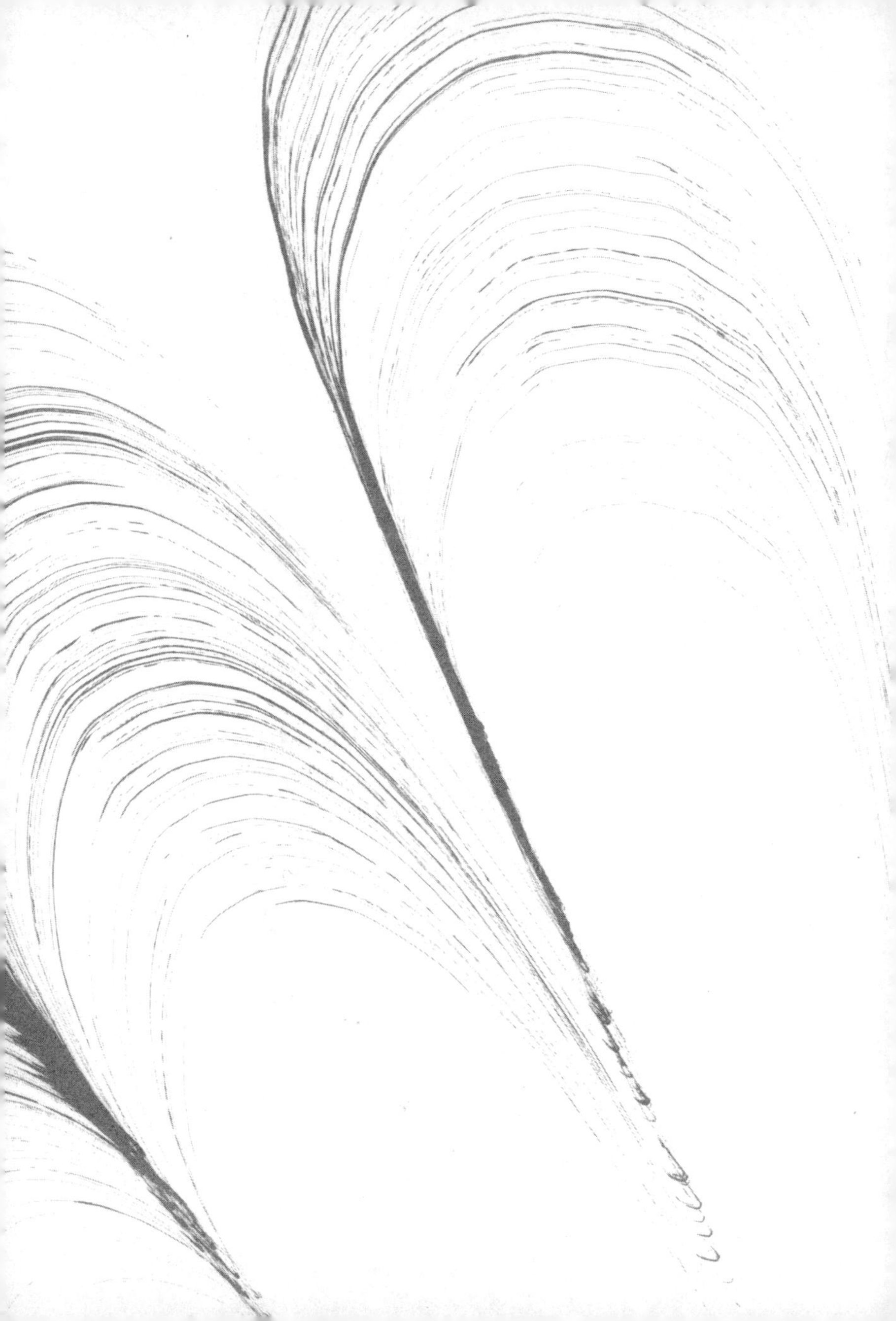

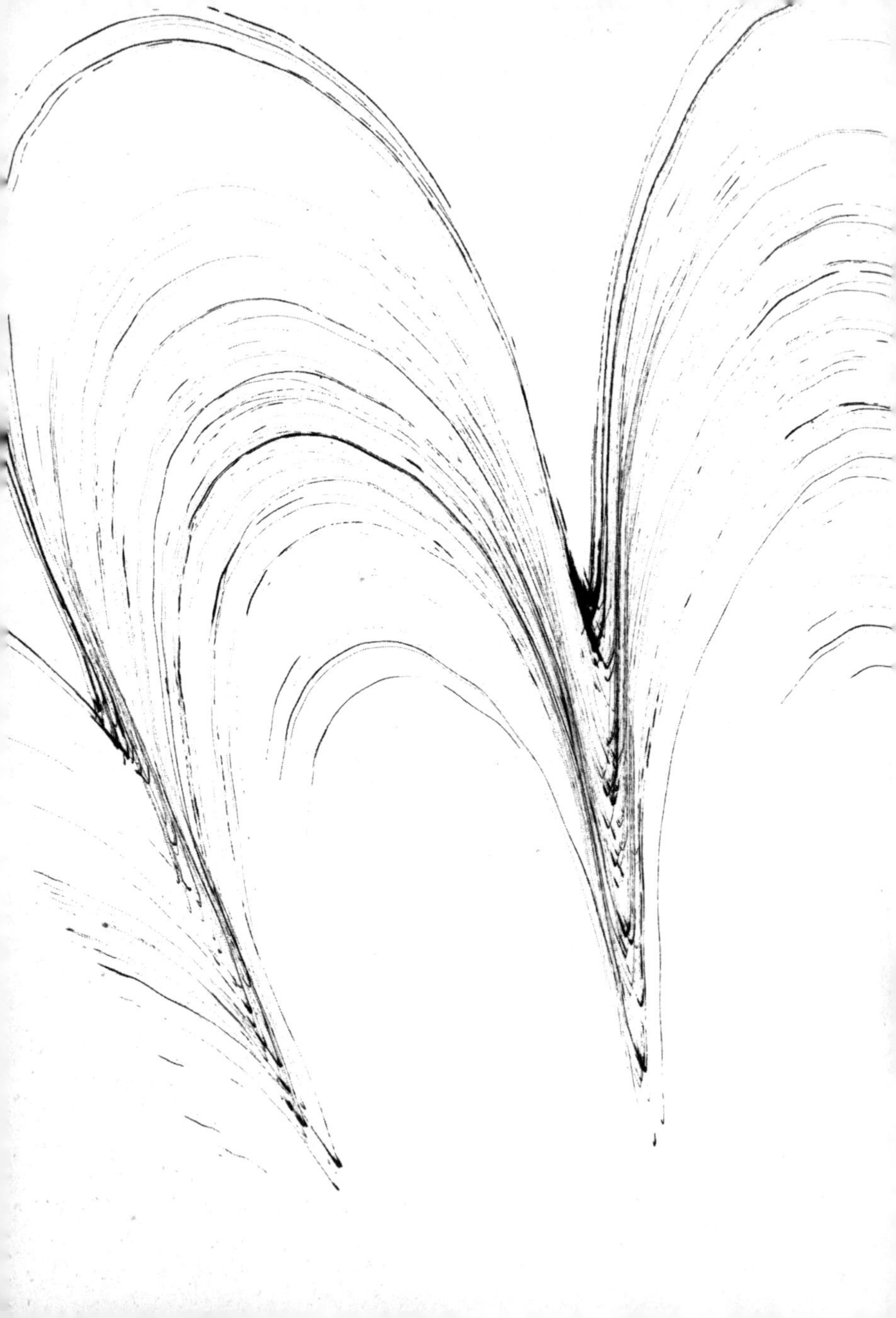

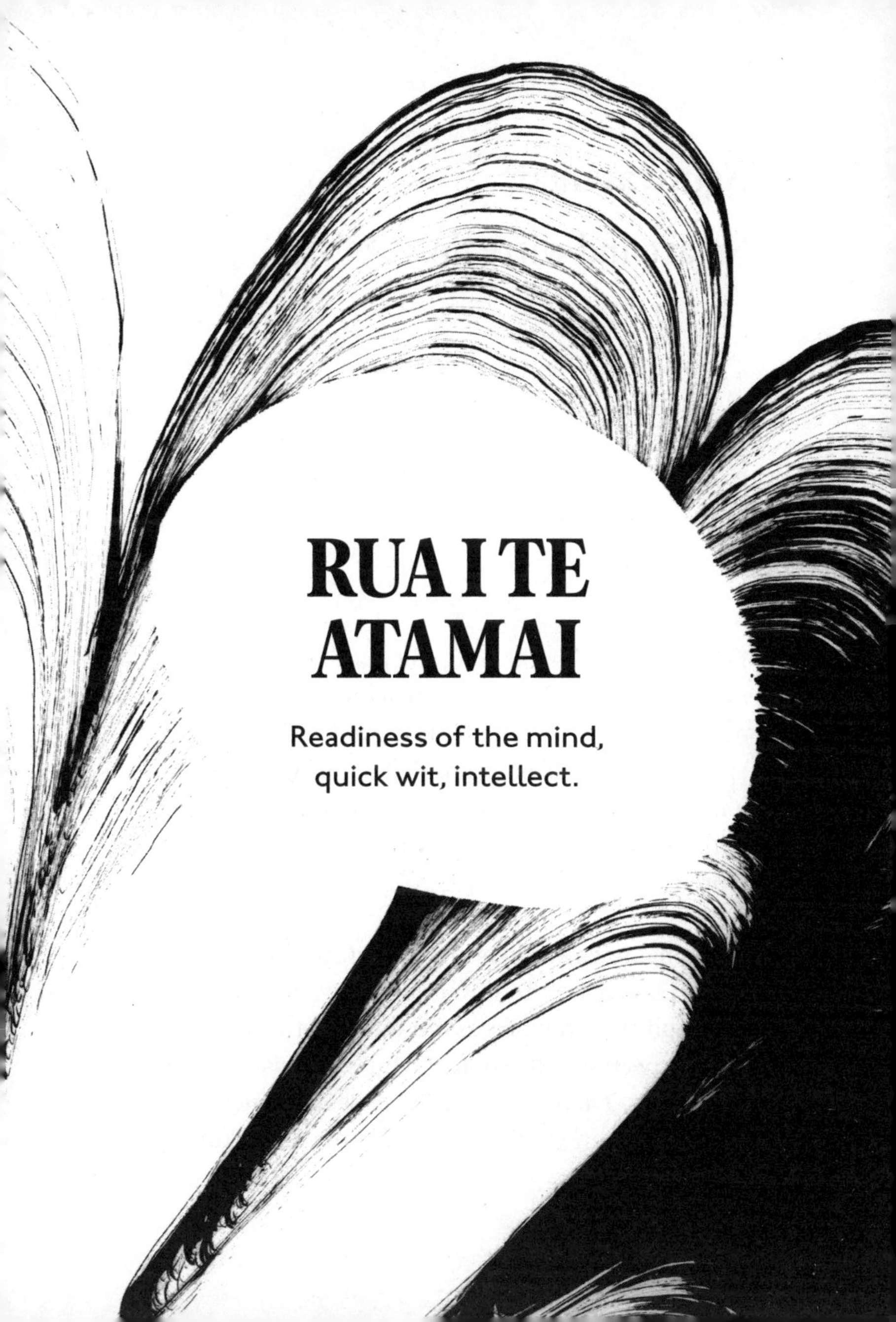

RUA I TE ATAMAI

Readiness of the mind, quick wit, intellect.

Ngutu atamai.

Smart and witty lips.

Leaving rua taketake o Io, the place of simplicity and stability, we have been reacquainted with our place in the incalculable expanse of time and space. We have been reminded of our tiny part in a much bigger story. We carry that ancient anchor with us. Now for a shift in what Hinengaro has stored up for us.

Stepping downwards into our next rua, we see lights playing on the surface of a wide pool of water. A lagoon stretches across our path. Not what we were expecting. The cool, playful water rises to lap at our feet. There is a dynamic expectant energy, a distinctive new challenge is ahead of us. Looking around we notice twinkling fairy-lights high above us, this is a friendly place. We can't help but smile. Stepping-stones map the only way to the other side. Some look to be slightly below the surface of the water. Immediately we can feel our internal analysis ramping up, working out how we might best navigate the crossing.

And there is no time to waste. Hinengaro compels us to move. We must jump from rock to rock. We feel the exhilaration as we leap from stone to stone. Despite all our internal computations, in the end, we must trust how Hinengaro integrates all of our possible responses.

Catching the surface of the pool, we kick water high into the air. It is as if the water sees the joke as the droplets circle above and then rain down again onto our upturned faces. A ready-made shower. A moment of fun. And at the same time Hinengaro demands our smartest moves. This is the territory of rapid response, of lightning-speed choices as she calls us to cross the expanse in record time.

I am reminded of the games we played at Te Hiku Okoro, our local language-revitalisation programme. Quick-fire hand-eye coordination, rhythmic claps and matching hand movements. Twisting around and back. Mental leaping from place to place, finding the confidence for quirky, even cheeky, replies. Rapid responses are what's needed. This is the essence of atamai. Our quick wit is such a central part of how Hinengaro works.

The speed of the banter shows the mental agility of the speaker. The perceptive comments that demonstrate the essence of atamai, the readiness of the mind, the intellect. A strong, adaptable and flexible resource is what we find waiting for us here.

Hinengaro makes us leap across the water in her own playful game. She shows us that we can practise these abilities and experience them with our whole being. And there is an emotional quality here too. Joy is part of our rua i te atamai; there is a pleasure in these activities that require mind-juggling, and this can lift everyone's spirits.

There is a famous story from Te Paatu, one of our local iwi, which exemplifies intelligence with a serious dose of wit. Mōroki and Koropeke were brothers who lived at Ōrūrū Pā, their stronghold. A Ngāpuhi war party had laid siege to the pā and resources inside were running low. The brothers sought advice from two tohunga, Te Au and Te Aratapu. How might it be possible to survive? These experts instructed that kete, baskets, must be woven, filled with soil, and finally be hung up in view of the marauding war party. The heavy kete didn't move in the wind, convincing the war party that those inside the pā had plenty of food. This smart thinking meant that the war party gave up and left. Those inside were now safe to collect food and plan their next moves. One of the first things they did was to tear down the huts Ngāpuhi had constructed for their siege. And they enshrined their own experience of atamai in the name of the iwi, the tribe. Known from then on as Te Paatu, reminding us of their act of destruction of the walls, the pātū, of the makeshift shelters left behind by the abandoned siege. A celebration of smart thinking, no doubt completed with a bit of 'e nge!', 'serves you right!'

Breathless and elated we reach the other side of the pool. Pausing here, we can begin to identify and build on our strengths in nimble thinking. Astute choices that lead to decisive, effective action. Brevity is inherent in this kind of quick thinking. Keeping it short and sweet. We can be confident enough to trust Hinengaro's unexpected lessons through playfulness.

What are some practical ways to build this flex as a whānau? Playing games together that involve everyone in some healthy competition, whether it is in sports, kapa haka, waka ama, card games, chess. Recognising that the savvy strategies we build together in everyday life have so much value. And they make living much more fun too.

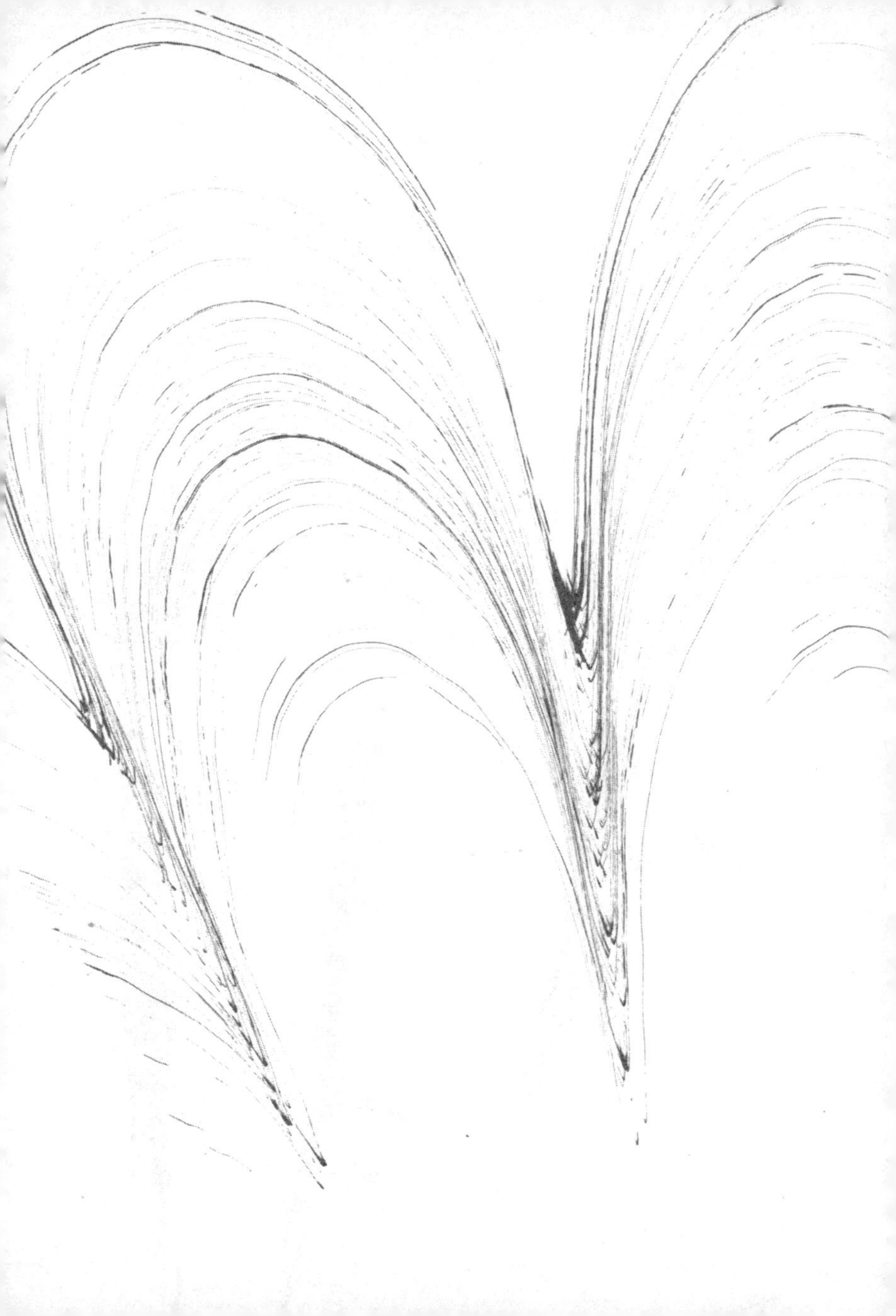

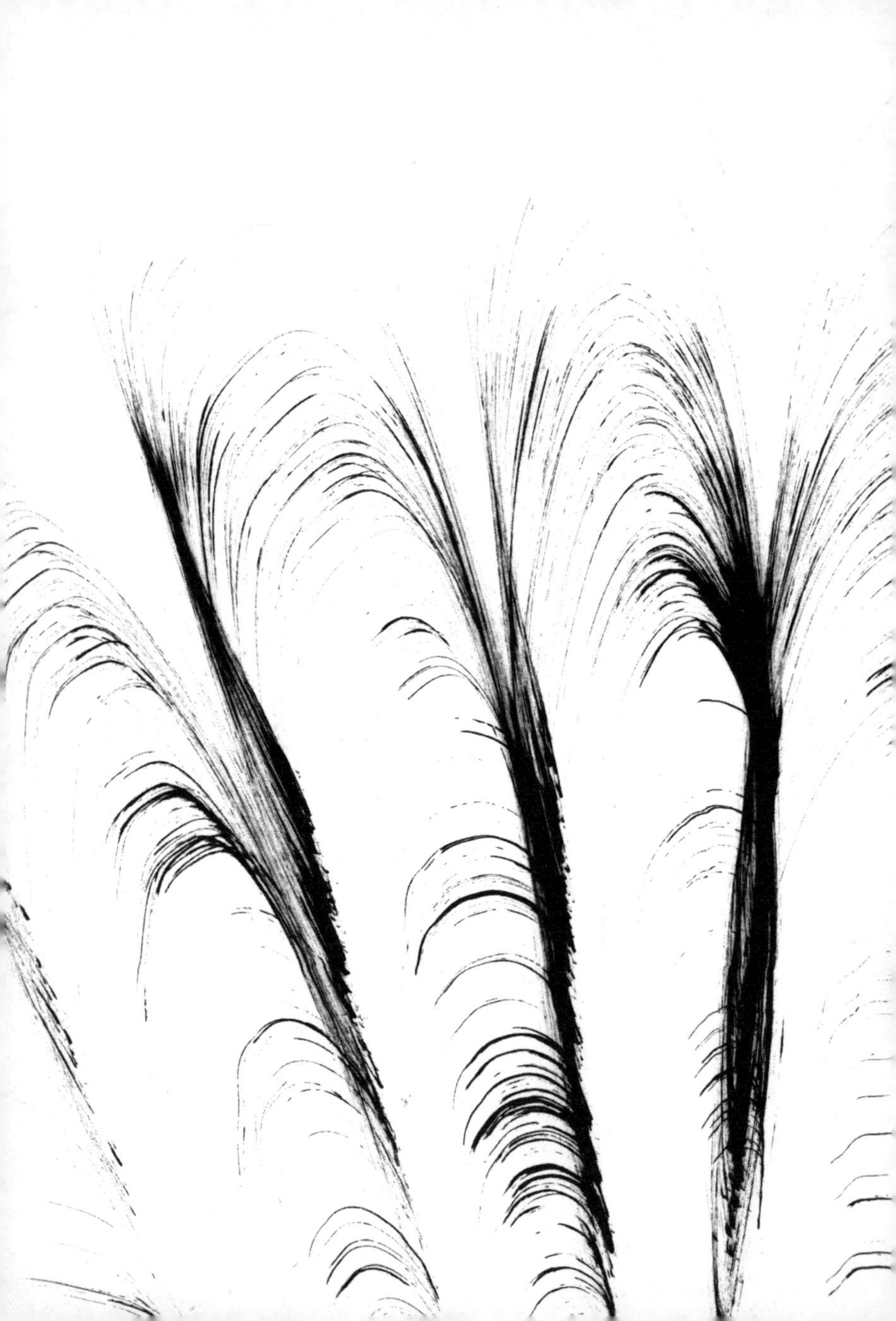

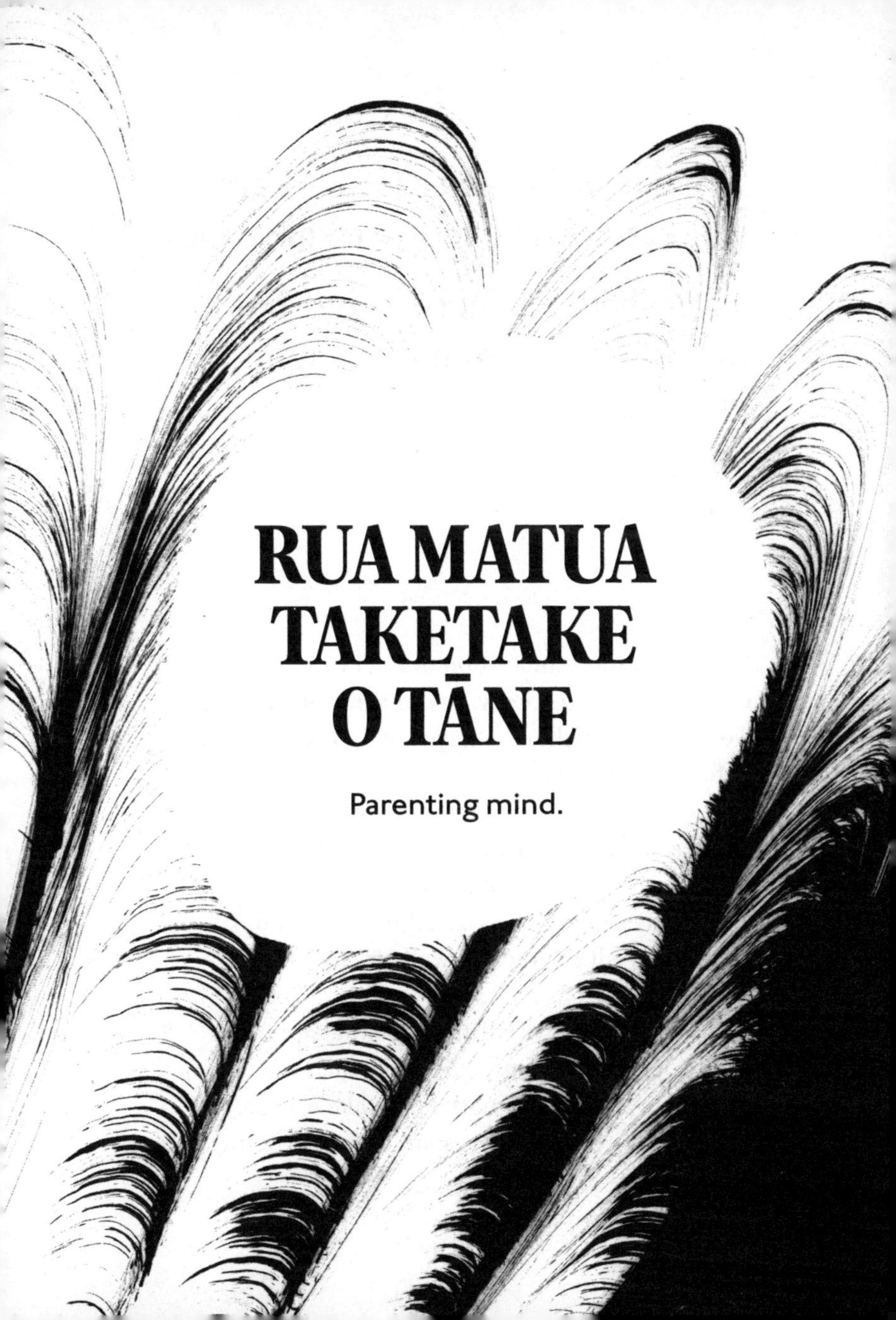

RUA MATUA TAKETAKE O TĀNE

Parenting mind.

‘Whakarua i te hau e taea te karo, whakarua i taku kōtiro e kore e taea.’

‘I can shelter from the wind, but I cannot shelter from the longing for my daughter.’

— Tōhē

Fuelled by the exhilaration of rua i te atamai, we now enter new territory. And it is no surprise that we are ready with our sharpened quick-thinking to enter our next rua.

Ledges form stairs leading upwards in a classic stepwise poutama formation. Here we face experiences of the need for adjustment and acceptance all around the walls of the cave.

This is a place of parenting. Our whakapapa, genealogy, is our focus, with this much-needed parenting angle. Rua matua taketake o Tāne. A unique place where the resources for parenting are stored. It should not surprise us that our ancestors recognised parenting as a fundamental aspect of Hinengaro's concerns. Without skilled and loving intergenerational parenting of our babies the tribe would die. Without thoughtful, confident and adaptable approaches to raising tamariki mokopuna in times gone by, the people would not have survived. Here in this rua we are dedicated to experiences of structured progress in our parenting and caregiving roles.

Poutama is our theme. Poutama is a well-recognised design from tukutuku panels and weaving. Repeated vertical lines rise up, with horizontal lines bending at a 90-degree angle, showing growth followed by a period of consolidation and a new equilibrium. This pattern continues over and over again, demonstrating periods of change followed by shaping a new state of being. In this rua, multiple shelves and steps jut out from the walls.

Messages of advancement and striving for improvement have been waiting for us in these rock staircases. It is an ancient language we recognise. Poutama depicts the way knowledge and skills add together, building on each other as we attain increasing levels of awareness, and with application of these skills we find a deepening spiritual connection to our caregiving roles.

Parenting is arguably one of the most demanding roles we ever take on. Over the course of our lives, we love and care for many tamariki, many children. We take responsibility for them now and into the future. It is fair to say that these modern times have put added and ever-changing pressure on all of us as parents and caregivers. Back in the days of our tūpuna, all adults were seen as parents, whether they had biological children or not. This is a useful reflection as we explore the steps around the walls. Circling around, we have a visceral sense of an earlier society centred on the needs of tamariki mokopuna. Thinking about them as parents of the future, learning by observation and by being included in discussions about parenting from the many parental figures who care for them.

As we walk up and down the poutama steps we gain different perspectives on the cave itself. The walls are warm to the touch and soft with a delicate springy moss. There is give and take here.

We breathe in the restorative atmosphere. Rejuvenating and at the same time restful.

I feel tears on my cheeks. This is a safe place to bring parenting fears and mistakes, to bring the strange painful growth we experience as parents, as caregivers. The parenting we learned from our own parents, and their parents before them. The distortions many of us experienced. The things we want to do differently. We often feel we are playing catch-up as the young ones pull ahead in their development. All of our negative self-talk comes out in this rua. We might have a harsh inner voice ringing in our ears, saying, 'no, not good enough'. How do we begin to support our young people with the difficulties of this era, so different from when we were young? This is the common theme we mull over as we traverse our poutama steps. Recriminations are released, bursting out into the void, to gradually find their silence, absorbed by the forgiving moss.

I have learned a lot from the journey into rua matua taketake o Tāne. I am so thankful that Hinengaro has this rua for a holistic intergenerational approach to our parenting in her cave vocabulary. She's practical, focusing on what really matters. As a child and adolescent psychiatrist, I am often working with parents in their own deep distress and fear about their tamariki. Many of our fathers find it difficult to express their feelings of loss of control. Their anger in the face of struggling with a sense of failure to heal their tamariki themselves. These dads often tell me how trapped they feel by their own pain. I have looked for ways to connect with our parents and those in parenting roles so we could begin to work together, and our parents might begin to trust us and themselves to find solutions.

Tōhē, one of our ancestors from Muriwhenua who lived at Maunga Piko, was a caring father. And a great chief. He is the one whom Te Oneroa a Tōhē, Ninety Mile Beach, is named after. His daughter Rāninikura had gone to live in a different area, on the Kaipara, and he missed her dearly. It is said that when he realised he was coming to the end of his life, he went to great lengths to try to see her. One of the things he is known to have said is, 'Whakarua i te hau e taea te karo, whakarua i taku kōtiro e kore e taea.' 'I can shelter from the wind, but I cannot shelter from the longing for my daughter.'

Tōhē's famous whakatauākī highlights how deep our love for our children runs, no matter what their age and stage. In a constructive and culturally meaningful way, this story of Tōhē helps build an honouring connection with our fathers in particular. And hence, better outcomes for our tamariki mokopuna on their life journeys.

Hinengaro leads us around her rua, helping us to discover our own openness to learn what could be most helpful in our roles as parents and caregivers. We can tune in to the ancient whispers of ngā pūkenga o mua, the experts of earlier times. We can find the patience to trust this learning, to follow in the footsteps of whakapapa, to be smart and to use our intelligence and wit. In this way, we can focus on the lessons that Hinengaro and her rua are highlighting.

What are some stories you can begin to discover when you spend time in this rua? Who can you bring to mind who is there to help you on your parenting and caregiving journey, to uncover what is available that resonates with you? Maybe people who have long passed, like Tōhē, who have left reminders of loving, nurturing parenting, and can be a source of inspiration? How can you map your own poutama of parenting? There are so many of your own stories already waiting for you here.

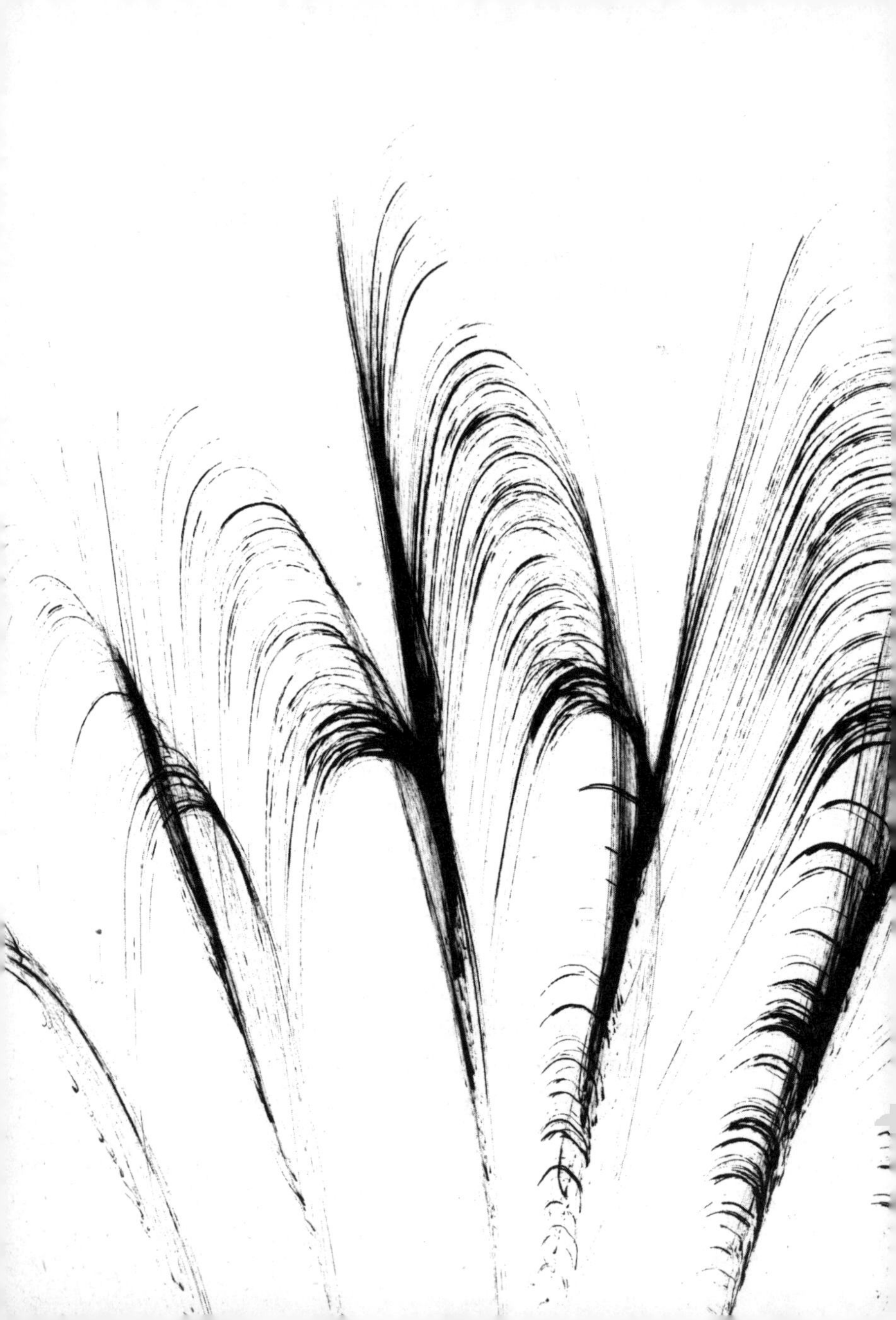

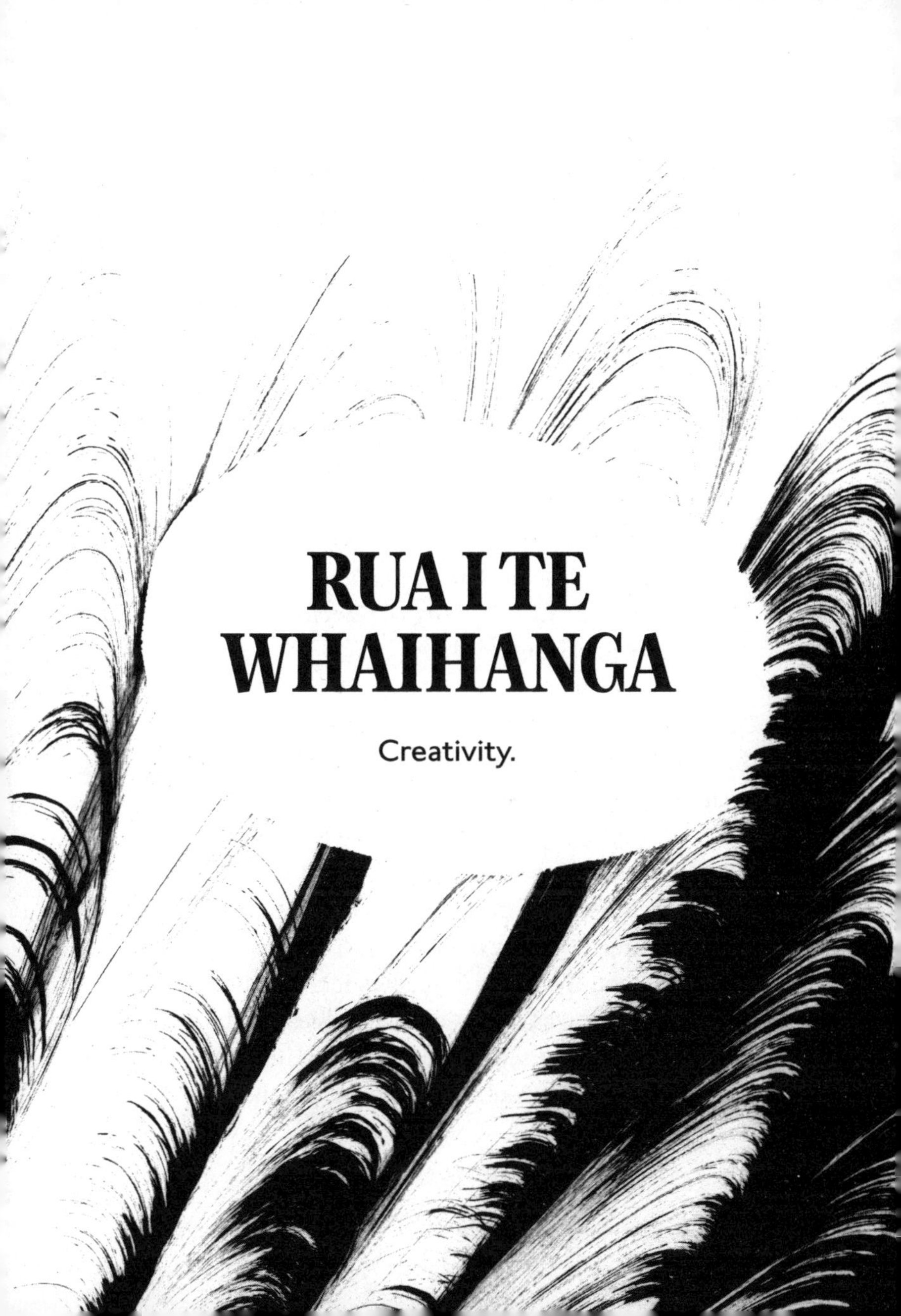

RUA I TE WHAIHANGA

Creativity.

E kōwhā ana a Hineteuira i tōna rua kanapu, i tōna rua kōhā.

Hineteuira lightning is flashing on her mountain peak.

There is a crackle of static on our skin. An electric charge ignites the air. Our hair stands on end. Hinekapua, our female deity of the clouds, is vigorously brushing our hair.

As we leave our rua matua taketake o Tāne, we find ourselves entering a place of swirling clouds, a rua with its own weather!

As the mist begins to lift, sparks crack with intensity. Electrons haka. Waves of adrenaline wash through us. Our eyes seem to stretch beyond their sockets. Even our eyelashes feel magnetised. The walls of the cave reveal themselves: multi-coloured rocks, hanging vines, the distinctive haunting notes of a kōauau, a tiny flute-like instrument.

A place dedicated to creativity.

Whenever we return here we feel a floating sensation, as if we are moving upwards with the mist, into the clouds where Hineteuira is birthing her baby lightning sparks. We feel such freedom of expression and the intense drive to create.

Hinengaro reminds us that we all have our own original source of creativity, our own whaihanga: literally the pursuit of creating, the activity of building.

In our rushing, distracted, overstimulated lives we can struggle to find our creativity. To rediscover the ease we had as youngsters in making a leaf and stick into a waka, in building a fort with cushions and a tarpaulin, scratching elaborate designs from our dreams into the wet sand.

Here Hinengaro has the assistance of Hinekapua and Hineteuira in providing the space to feel the inner lightning bolts that drive us to express our creativity. The mists begin with a shrouding effect, the path is unclear, cloaked in mystery. Here we can bring our so-called 'writer's block', our having no idea about what to cook for dinner, or when we are feeling seriously lacking in motivation, to rediscover the surge and flash of our own creative urges.

Hinengaro reminds us that mists lift. And that even the air contains such powerful forces of electrical charge. Hinengaro shows us her forceful energy through the sparks she provides in our brains and hearts, in our skin.

We have all been to see some creative activities that we found profoundly inspiring. *Whakapaupākihi* is a unique performance blending haka and musical theatre about the exploits of three brothers from Te Tai Rāwhiti that stays with me. An extraordinary bilingual whānau developed and produced this reimagining of their own ancestors' stories. Those of us privileged enough to see the performances have been forever changed by them. Such is the power of creativity.

We all have creativity within us. We don't have to be the most skilled speaker, artist, musician, singer or performer. Or the epitome of creativity in sporting prowess. Or as a kaiako, teacher. Or be the ultimate in our creative approach to mahinga kai, gardening, or as cooks. Hinengaro invites us to recognise our own creativity in our own spheres, in our own lives.

How does being in rua i te whaihanga affect you? It can be very full-on at first. It can make us feel useless and inadequate. Let's linger. Maybe we can hear an inner voice, one that comes from long ago, telling us we are not creative, as we wait? Resist the urge to rush ahead because we feel a little uncomfortable. Allow the initial awkwardness to drift away with the clouds. Then we begin to notice a shift. We are born creative. We have creativity running through our veins. Now we can let those old beliefs float away. Let those old ideas explode into a million pieces with the power of lightning bolts.

Creative expression is our birthright. How can you be purposeful in your curiosity to rediscover your creative talents? You could harness the power of Māui, the great mischief-maker and rule-breaker. And you don't have to take it to Māui's extremes. No one is expecting you to slow down the sun like he did. And yet, here is a designated place, a rua where you can put yourself in Māui's shoes and imagine how that would feel. Hot work slowing down Tamanuiterā, the sun! And you never know, once Hinengaro has helped you to brainstorm Māui's exploits in this rua, you may find you have unlocked a whole raft of brave, creative solutions for the current challenges in your life.

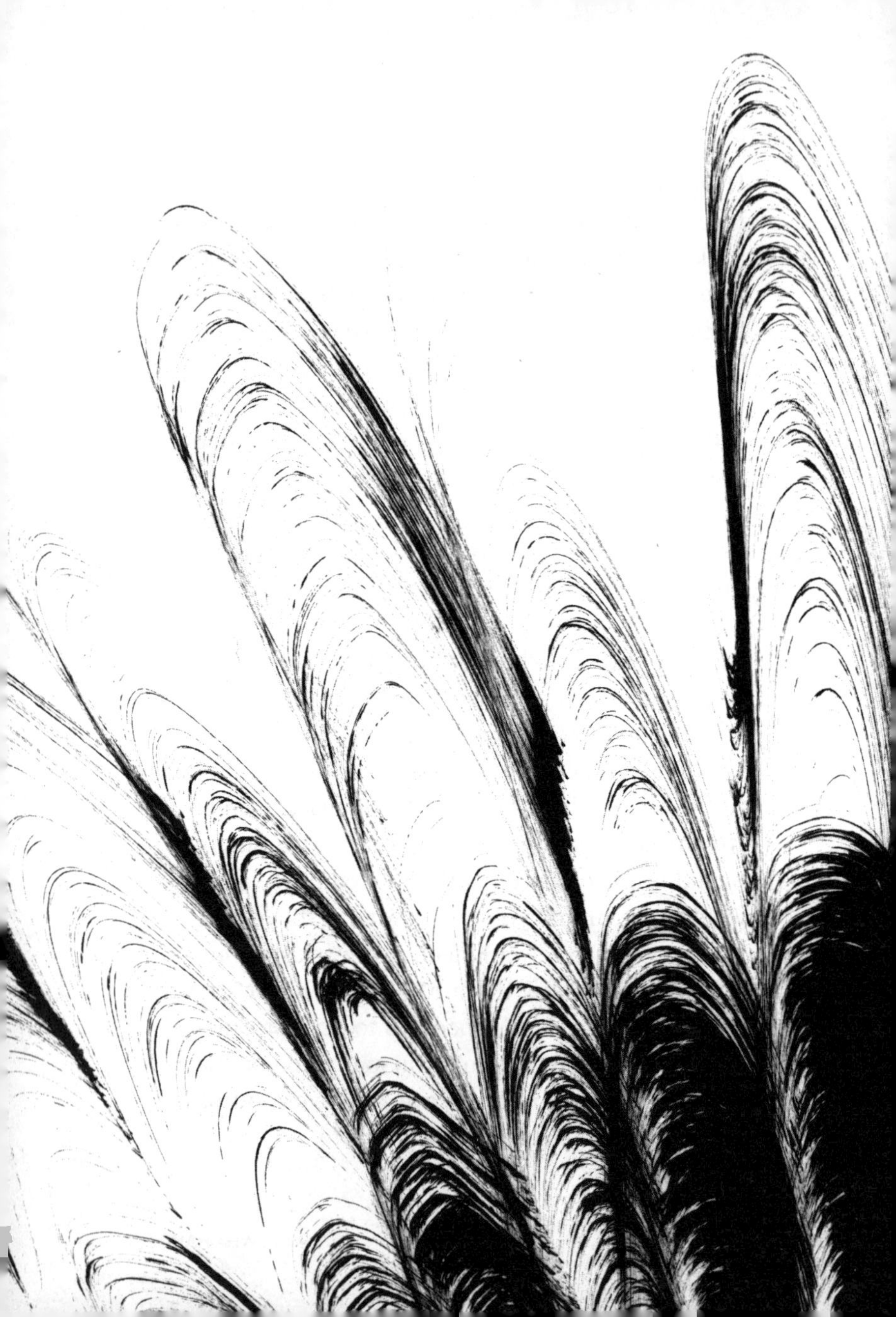

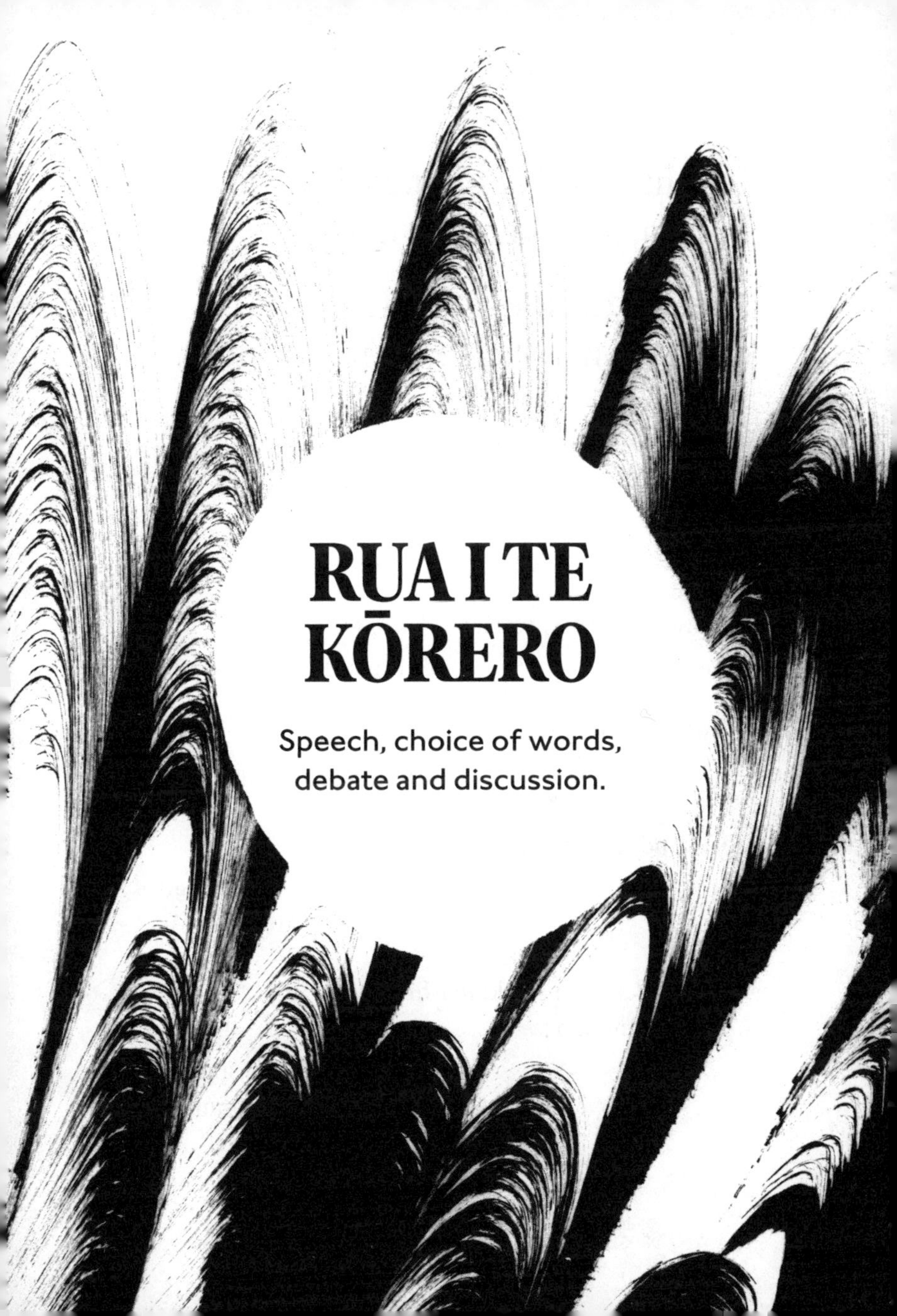

RUA I TE KŌRERO

Speech, choice of words, debate and discussion.

He aha te kai a te rangatira? He kōrero, he kōrero, he kōrero.

What is the food of chiefs? It is discussion, it is debate, it is oratory.

Te Kawariki, Te Kawariki

Te Kawariki, Te Kawariki

Tirotiro kau noa kei hea

examining carefully where

Te iwi, nōna ngā tapuwae e whāia nei

the footsteps of those who lead,
are taking us

Rere whakateuru atu ki te tihi
o Whangatauatia

fly to the west, to the summit
of Whangatauatia

Mā te one i haea ai e Pōroa

to the beach on which Pōroa
drew the line

Heoi kāhore kau i reira

but, no not there

Huri whakaterāwhiti atu ki Pūwheke

we turn to the east to Pūwheke

Mā te moana a Rangaunu me ōna pioke e

to the ocean of Rangaunu
and their pioke

Heoi kāhore kau i reira

but no, not there either

Ū ana te mata ki muri

face steadfastly to the north, the place
of departed spirits

Ki ngā wai pūataata o Pārengarenga

to the clear waters of Pārengarenga

Ki te ara ka rere kore ki muri

to the path of no return

Ki te whakatōreretanga o te wairua

to the place where wairua leaps away

Ki Te Rēinga e

to Te Rēinga

Koia ahau te whakataukī e

indeed, I am represented by
this proverbial saying

Tēnā a Te Kawariki

namely, Te Kawariki

Me whakapakari e.

that is what must strengthen me.*

~

Hinengaro welcomes us from the intensity of rua i te whaihanga straight into rua i te kōrero.

How fitting! Creatively restored, reignited, we can approach kōrero, what we say, from that enriched sense of being. Here, inside the cave,

* Jones, S. (1984). *Te Kawariki*, Muriwhenua.

we see the shapes of many peaks and ridges. Some are humble mounds, just an easy stride to their summits. Others are majestic, with steep slopes defying any attempt to scale them. A cave filled with its own landscape of rocky knolls and hillocks.

The pepeha we have begun with, a famous tribal narrative, Te Kawariki, lives and breathes the power of kōrero. Straddling the peaks of our mountains and hills, the various aspects of the stories of Muriwhenua.

What is Te Kawariki? Like many aspects of te ao Māori, Te Kawariki can be many things, all at the same time. As we are fond of saying, 'iti te kupu, nui te kōrero', 'a few words, with a lot of layers'. Te Kawariki can be a plant with berries, eaten to foster resilience; it can be a lizard; and it can be an indigenous yellow parrot. Te Kawariki was also the name of a group formed in Te Hiku o te Ika, the Far North, to fight for and invigorate our treasured language and histories for generations to come. This group, Te Kawariki, composed this pepeha. Embedded in the words is an innate confidence about our collective future, a place in time yet to come, where our descendants of the future live.

This story-telling device, using the flight of Te Kawariki traversing our sacred places, reminds us where we come from. This portable cultural technology is our cultural calling card. A carefully constructed story locating us in our Indigenous continuum. A continuum not only in this current world, but also our world across time and space.

Hinengaro ensures that this kōrero gives us the means to go back and forth, through past, present and future, and to visit these sacred vantage points, all while remaining right here. This Māori time travel is how we identify, how we reaffirm who we are.

Here in this rua we are filled with the power of kōrero. In this rua we feel ourselves become part of ngā maunga whakahī, puke kōrero; uplifting mountains, hills that hold our stories. They are our sources of kōrero, keepers of these precious tools. And we carry them with us wherever we go.

Te Kawariki references many stories, many taonga, many treasures which are inherently linked together. This kōrero serves as a concise, nuggety form of story, the purpose of which is to reaffirm who we are. Strengthening connectivity is a key purpose of our choice of words. Bringing back into the front of our minds who we are through these taonga, these treasures of many kinds. By speaking the names of these people and places out loud we keep their stories alive, we keep them warm. We show our love and care for them. We bring forward how precious they are for future generations. This kōrero is an essential part of our identity. These words are embedded in how we understand the life lessons of our lands and ancestors. This is how we see our place in the world.

When we speak in te reo Māori, we all feel the unique vibration of our language. This language in itself is part of the time-travel portal too. When we speak our own language, speak our words out loud, our phrases, using the language of our old people, we open up our connections with them. Our reo opens us up to the dreams of our old people. Their plans for us, going back thousands of years. From our ancestors, through us, and on to those who come after us, these stories weave our lines of whakapapa, our genealogy, with each other and the universe. Greeting each other from the knowledge that we are ancestors of the future, we welcome our own dreams and plans for our descendants.

We feel these reo vibrations with our wairua. Wairua, the fundamental basis of our wellbeing, our connection with everything in the universe. Our deep spiritual awareness of being is also experienced as our intuition, what we sense in the pit of our gut. We continue to carry that intense, expansive awareness of wairua from our very first rua, rua i te horahora, throughout Hinengaro's cave ride.

Hinengaro transports us to those places to be with our wheinga when reciting our histories. We stand in those places with our ancestors, on the peaks of their mountain tops. These narratives enable me to bring you along too. We can travel in time and space together.

These stories also outline the requirements, the necessities handed down from our tūpuna. They are an instruction manual for life, holding medicinal properties. He rongoā tō te kōrero, kōrero is medicine. These phrases and metaphors tell us how and where to find who we are. They give us a blueprint for our wellbeing.

Everyday work shows me a persistent lack of wellbeing in our communities. And the huge potential for change. It is no wonder that we are all, in our own ways, struggling to recognise what our own true wellbeing might be when most of us have had to relearn our own language. Many of our parents and grandparents were beaten for speaking te reo Māori at school. Re-learning our kōrero is reclaiming our identity. Along the way the intergenerational losses and grief come to the surface. It is emotional. It hurts.

Without knowing the kōrero, without knowing the stories, without knowing the taonga that come to life in our stories, we suffer profound loss and grief. Losses without names or validation. Because how do you name the grief and loss of the language, stories and taonga of ancestors you don't even know?

We are not alone. Many peoples across the world face similar intergenerational hurt and pain. They are facing these same losses and the fight to reclaim their stories. Reclaiming all of our healthy narratives means going back many generations. This kōrero has so many layers, no matter our cultural backgrounds. Within these stories are the keys to understanding the old ways of being part of the natural world. These are stories we need to include in our fight for climate justice, for solutions that work for us.

Reclaiming our own kōrero means we can navigate our own migration home to our identity as kaitiaki, as guardians. To all the ways to express our humanity, to express being Māori. Like Te Kawariki, the tireless birds who carry our stories on high, through all kinds of weather, to land where it is safe, and share kōrero over and over again from one generation to the next.

The words we choose and how we put them together have such potent meaning and so much potential for what we need in our world right now. Indigenous stories carry ancient insight and action for the changes we need, that are so relevant on our chaotic planet. These stories speak about a very different relationship with our world, living in respectful reciprocity with Papatūānuku, our Mother Earth. These stories have the power to inspire and activate people from around the globe. To replenish the depleted energies and tired stories that are no longer relevant in the face of our planetary emergencies.

We have witnessed stories being used to try to drown out and dominate others. The louder voices, with more power and money, continue to be in control of many of the global stories. Here is a place to reflect on our choices of words and how we might unwittingly become a mouthpiece for stories that belong to others. How can we ensure we are not being pitted against our own people, guarding against the possibility of lateral violence? Hinengaro demands we examine the quality of the words we choose to tell our stories, and to be vigilant about how we interpret the stories we are exposed to.

What can we learn from spending time in rua i te kōrero? How can we be more mindful of our own kōrero, internally and with others? Words can so easily become weapons. Remember our whakataukī, 'He tao rākau ka taea te karo, he tao kī e kore e taea.' 'The thrust of a spear can be avoided, but not a tongue lashing.' Words can hurt. And those words and the pain they caused can stay with us. Conversely, words can also provide comfort and encouragement. The reassurance conveyed in the saying, 'Kaua e mate wheke, me mate ururoa!' 'Never give up, be like a hammerhead shark!'

How will you work on your choice of words and the stories they tell after spending time in rua i te kōrero? What could you do when you realise your words are hurtful, are causing pain? How can you let others know when you recognise your words were the wrong words? Let Hinengaro help you to choose better words to find your own voice and your own story.

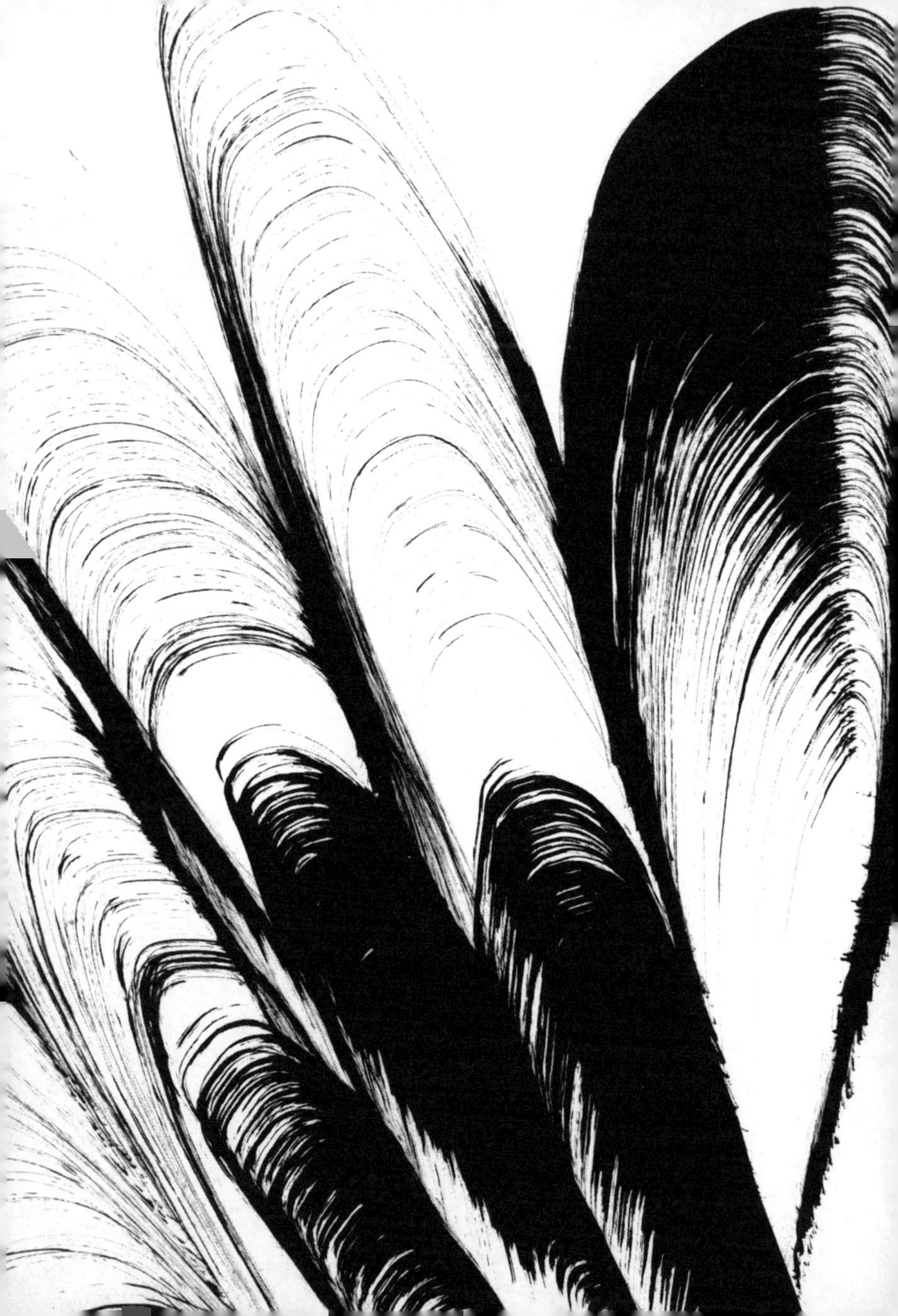

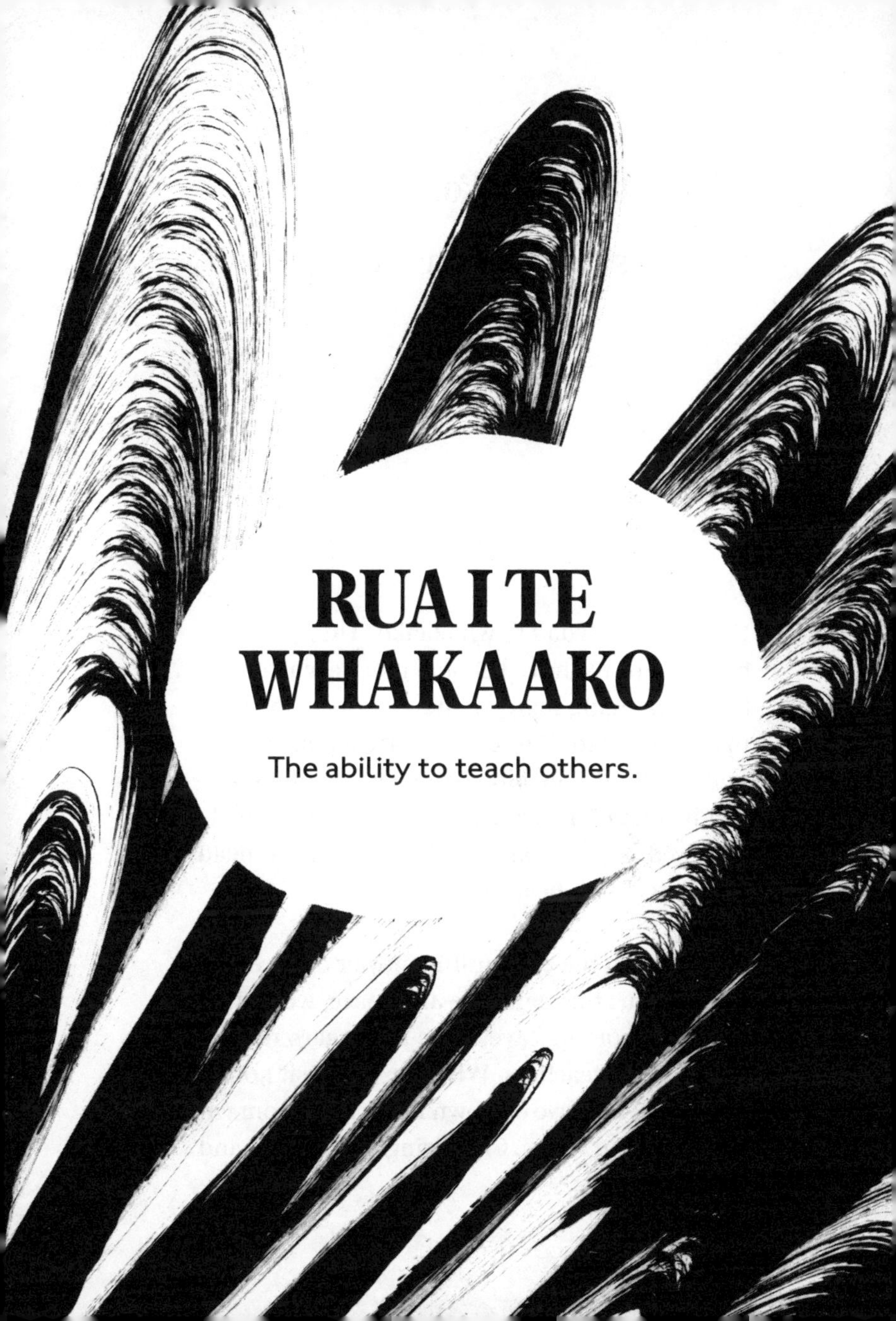

RUA I TE WHAKAAKO

The ability to teach others.

Tū ana hei Pouako.

Stand as teachers in life.

Nau mai ki te rua i te whakaako. Things are hotting up. We have become more accustomed to the changing light; we have come to expect the unexpected. We sense we are a long way underground. The blood-red earth under our feet is warm. The iron ore is visible in the rust-coloured sedimentary rock walls. Our foreheads are dotted with beads of sweat.

Moving with the exhilarating power of kōrero to transport us through time and space, we arrive at this welcoming cave. Here Hinengaro reminds us we are all teachers. Whether we like it not. For one thing, we have our own inner classroom where we school ourselves. Chastising our failures and probably not celebrating our successes as much as we could do.

Our ability to teach others is deeply impacted by our own experiences of being taught. For many of us, school was a mixed bag. For many there was conflict about how our names were pronounced, or we were renamed by teachers who refused to say our real names. Or we were not offered subjects we wanted to pursue. We feel those hot tears of school humiliation and shame. And yet there were also the unforgettable teachers who nurtured us and became such a positive part of our life stories.

One of the aspects of Te Hiku Okoro, our local reo programme in Muriwhenua, has been the premise that we are all teachers, whether we hold a qualification or not. Having whānau members and certified teachers learning together is a brilliant strategy, building such rich cohesion and appreciation for the benefits of unlocking our collective teaching skills. Ensuring that communication and skill-sharing between home and school keeps us all vibrant and inspired. Holding our tamariki mokopuna in such a healthy net, all of us committed to teaching and learning in all corners of our communities.

Recognising we are teaching ourselves and others all the time can feel alarming and even paralysing. We can become afraid to do anything for fear of teaching the wrong thing. Truly seeing that every aspect of our lives is a potential teaching moment for others, especially those we love, can feel overwhelming. Seeing how we can be much more deliberate in the process and content of what we want to teach is extremely challenging.

Are we teaching our babies that some emotions are acceptable, and others are not? Are we teaching, with subtle or overt cues, ways to express who we are that are preferred and others that we punish? Even when we believe that we are not teaching judgement and exclusion, maybe we are. And when this is pointed out, how defensive do we become?

Here in this nurturing cavern of teaching riches, we can relax and feel safe to let Hinengaro take us around all our fears about what we are teaching and how we can improve. 'Pai tū, pai hinga', which can be translated as 'It's good to try, it's good to fail'. Many of us have been taught to actively avoid any risk of failing, haven't we? Here Hinengaro reinforces that mistakes are an important part of the teaching–learning energies.

I remember one of our pouako at a kura reo began a lesson describing how he had failed by talking too long as the leader of his kapa in a competition. Points were deducted and the team lost. It was a powerful lesson coming from an esteemed teacher. His sharing his own sense of failure, of letting others down, helped to relieve a lot of tension in our own learning. If he could admit his mistakes and learn from them, so could we.

We know that the best, most effective teachers inspire us, that they take their time to get to know us. They have unwavering patience. They care. Maybe you can think of teachers in your life who made you feel you could learn and achieve. These teachers are so precious.

For those of us who are not officially teachers, recognising our roles as teachers, with the ability to teach valuable lessons in life, is an important moment too.

Here in rua i te whakaako we feel the blood, sweat and, no doubt, some tears about the process of learning and teaching. What do we want to teach ourselves? What do we want to teach others? What and how do we best learn, and learn to teach? What is the legacy of teaching and learning that we want to leave behind?

In our reo, teaching and learning have the same word: 'ako'. Ako speaks to the unique reciprocity of these experiences. An acknowledgement that the teacher and student are both learning and both teaching at the same time. How can you put the concept of whakaako into practice in your daily life? What can Hinengaro's rua of whakaaro provide to help you in your quest to teach and learn for a better life?

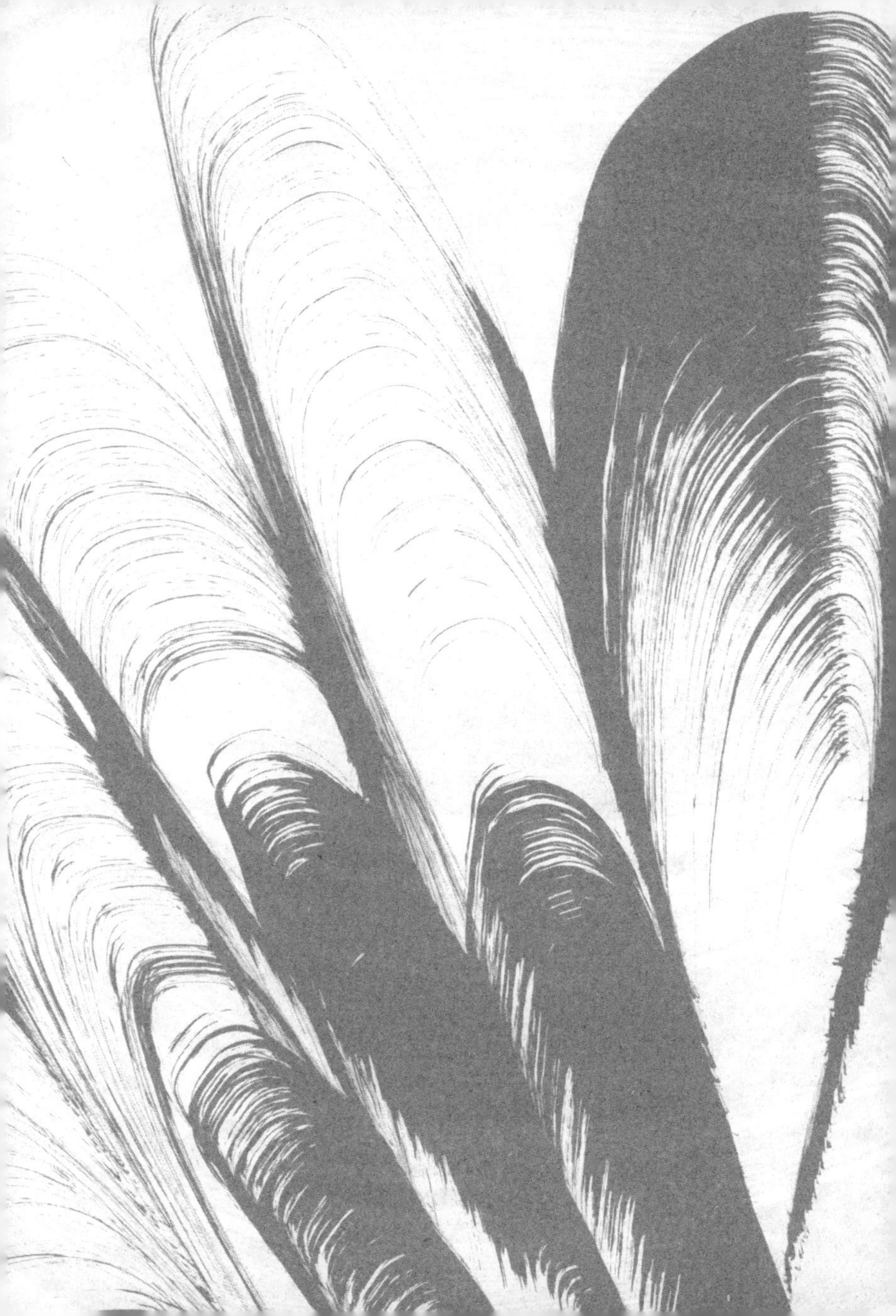

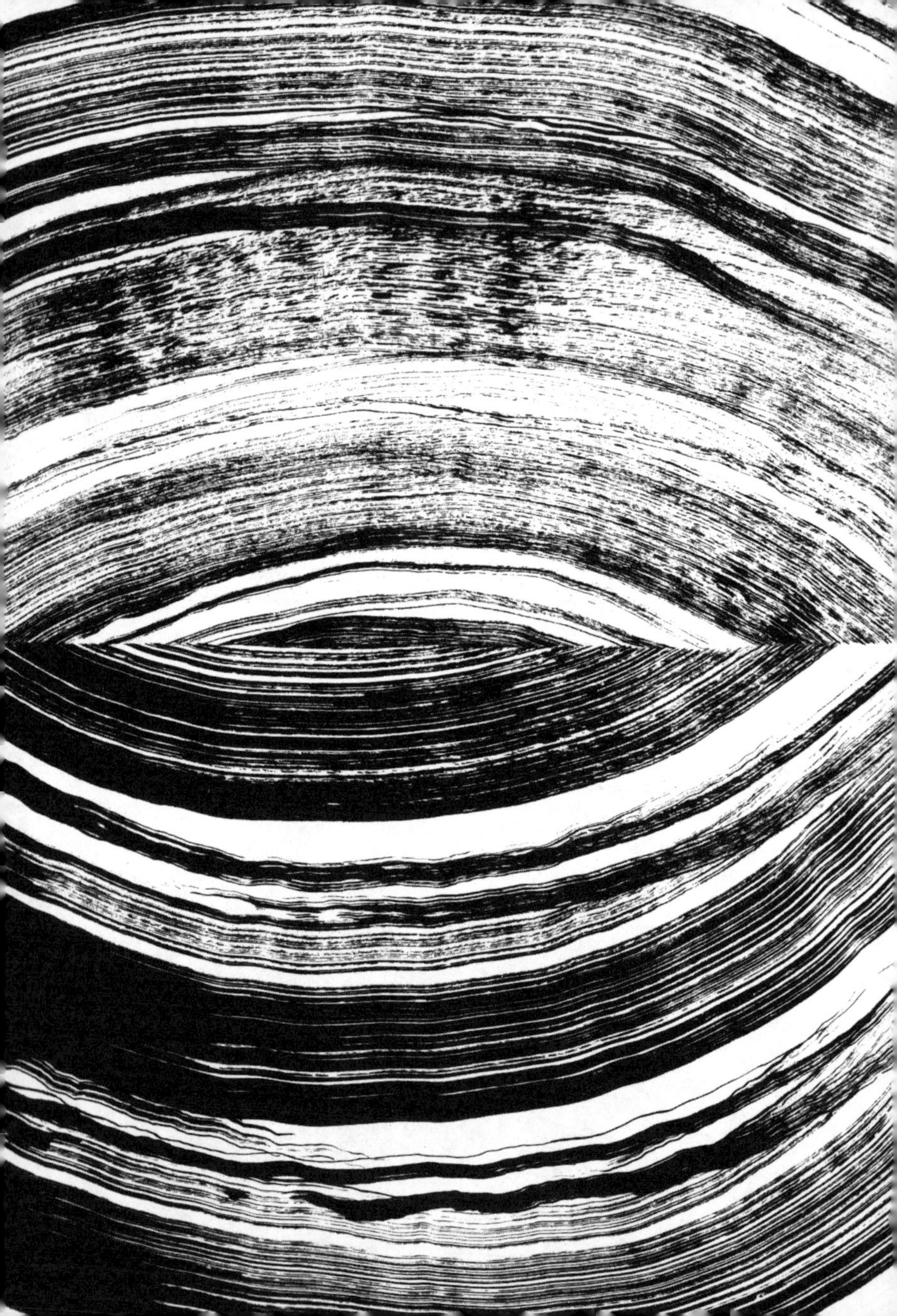

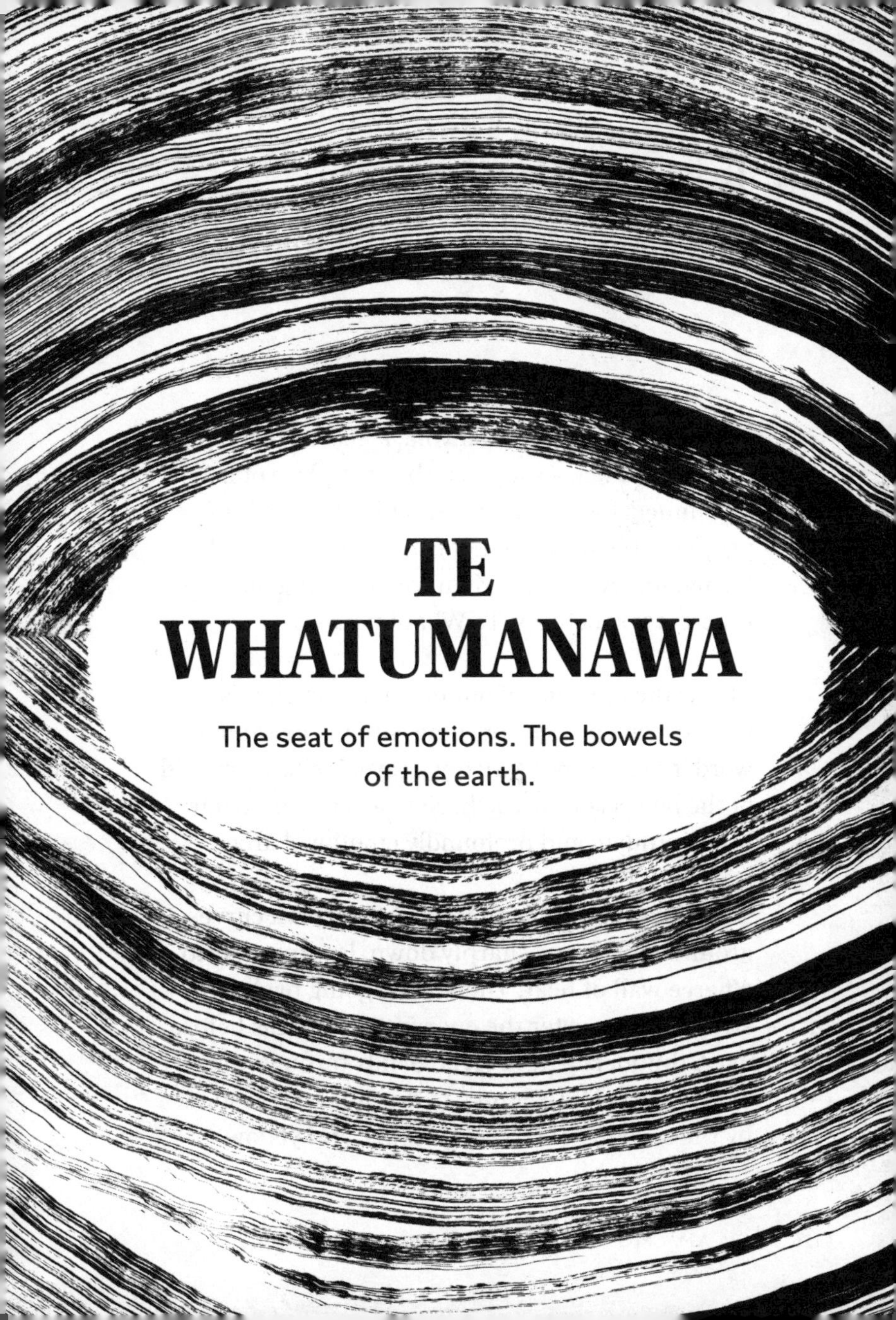

TE WHATUMANAWA

The seat of emotions. The bowels of the earth.

Te kūao maha a Araiteuru.

The many offspring of Araiteuru.

Araiteuru is a famous taniwha, a guardian creature from Hokianga, a sacred harbour. A place of new beginnings for our wheinga. A birthplace of our people in the north. Hinengaro returns me to the formidable Araiteuru when when visiting our innermost sanctuary, Te Whatumanawa.

This is the only one of our destinations on this journey which does not come with the precursor word 'rua'. It is not actually a cave. We have arrived at the bowels of the earth. Now we set foot in our most intimate and profoundly emotional arena.

The warmth rapidly intensifies. Our path curves around and slopes sharply down, leading us into a fierce wall of heat. There is no going back. We struggle to register the enormity of what is before us. A thundering lava river grinds through the chasm far below. Chunks of crushed rock jostled by the streams of dazzling orange and yellow.

Flames spiking up from the serpentine body of living fire. The tang of smoke and heat. Nostrils flaring, we check for a safe place to stand, bearing witness to the power of Te Whatumanawa. We are in the depths of Papatūānuku. The crucible of emotion. Hinengaro has created this terrifying place for us to recognise the wellspring of passion that we all have inside.

The power of emotion floods us. The proximity to danger, to imminent risk. The power to destroy so close at hand. And yet Hinengaro also provides this vantage point that allows us to experience this.

What does it mean that Hinengaro brings us so close to the very edge of our own thundering flow of molten rock? Hinengaro shows us that our deepest feelings have the power to melt stones, to cause mountains to move. Our big feelings: rage, fear, anger, lust, love and shame. Our inner taniwha, like the terrifying Araiteuru and her whānau, her extended family.

Te Whatumanawa is a place to come to stand in the blast furnace of our own feelings and to begin to recognise what they are about. Where that lava flow comes from and where it is heading. Hinengaro reminds us that we can use our emotions to redirect this driving relentless flow at any time. We can find healthy ways to express these ancient feelings and release the fear of them taking control of our lives.

Our emotions are another superpower. They shape our perspective. They shift our position. They change our course. Hinengaro gives us the opportunity to feel what it is like inside the flow of lava. Te Whatumanawa gives us eyes of fire. From inside the waves of smelted rock we can sense the fearful radiance of all our emotions. How alive does this make us feel to be swept up in the current, within the tide of the flames surging around us? Here we can be renewed, forever changed. We grow in these flames. Our emotions, our desires are unashamedly raw. Te Whatumanawa is the cardiovascular system of our decisions and plans. The oxygen and the pumping emotional blood flow of our lives.

We have had to work hard to get all the way down here. Hinengaro has taken us through the first half of her pilgrimage. We have traversed to this depth, bringing with us lessons from the all-encompassing vision of wairua, the thrill in learning, recognition of the skills we need to keep expanding, and our powerful memory. She has led us through storehouses of patient growth in our learning, and the stripping away of distraction to find the simplicity of Io, guiding us to our own tao waka, our own ballast. Hinengaro has chased us across the wide pool of rua i te atamai, demanding quick thinking and wit; she has shown us the progression of our parenting mindset and the layers of creativity as the mists lift and the lightning crackles. Hinengaro has brought us deep into the heart of our mountains with the time and space travel that kōrero manifests, and has helped us to embrace the blood, sweat and tears of our teaching abilities. Now we are sweltering in the pit of unfiltered emotion. Hinengaro helps us to let go of fear, to stand and absorb all of our raw emotions raging below.

We are emotional beings. We feel things. Somehow this world tries to shape us as if we don't have emotions, or at least tells us that we should keep our emotions tightly under control. So that when our feelings spill out of our eyes and mouths and hearts, it is our fault, we are labelled weak, we are to blame, we are not normal.

Our tangihanga, traditional funeral practices, are such powerful expressions of emotion. We sob, we wail, we let the snot run down our faces. We are contorted with grief and loss. This is expected. This is normal for us. We struggle with funerals where people seem to try to hide their tears. That is a different cultural norm.

Hinengaro asks us the question, when emotions feel awkward or out of place, how can we find a way to express them safely? How can we help tamariki mokopuna, our children and grandchildren, trust that their feelings can be expressed and embraced, valued, and learned from?

Some people have found going to the top of a hill and screaming at the top of their lungs helps to let off steam. Others use the body to work off rage, fear and traumatic pain by playing contact sports, lifting weights, dancing, practising jiu-jitsu. We all need to find a safe way to ensure that we utilise what we learn about ourselves in Te Whatumanawa. Hinengaro will not allow us to shy away from this for long before the energy of our liquified emotional core erupts.

What can you do while you spend some time in Te Whatumanawa? What neatly tucked-away feelings are beginning to melt?

Taniwha, powerful guardians, emerge from their lairs when it is safe and they are ready to explore. Taniwha can be cautious about when they come out into the open as others may want to hunt them down and destroy them. Like our ancient taniwha, our powerful emotions sometimes make us feel fierce and indestructible. And we might not always be aware when our emotional reactions frighten or hurt others. You may have experienced other people trying to shut down your feelings sometimes, making your emotions burst out with even more power. Maybe you are becoming aware that some of your emotions make you feel out of control? Here is a safe place to discover your very own taniwha of Te Whatumanawa. How can you maximise the benefits? How can you share what you experience here in Te Whatumanawa with others to learn how your emotional experiences shape how you see your life, your relationships, your work and your future? Hinengaro brings us to Te Whatumanawa to show us that this is being human. This is something we all share. How can visiting Te Whatumanawa help you to grow different ways of knowing how the lava-hot emotions flow within you?

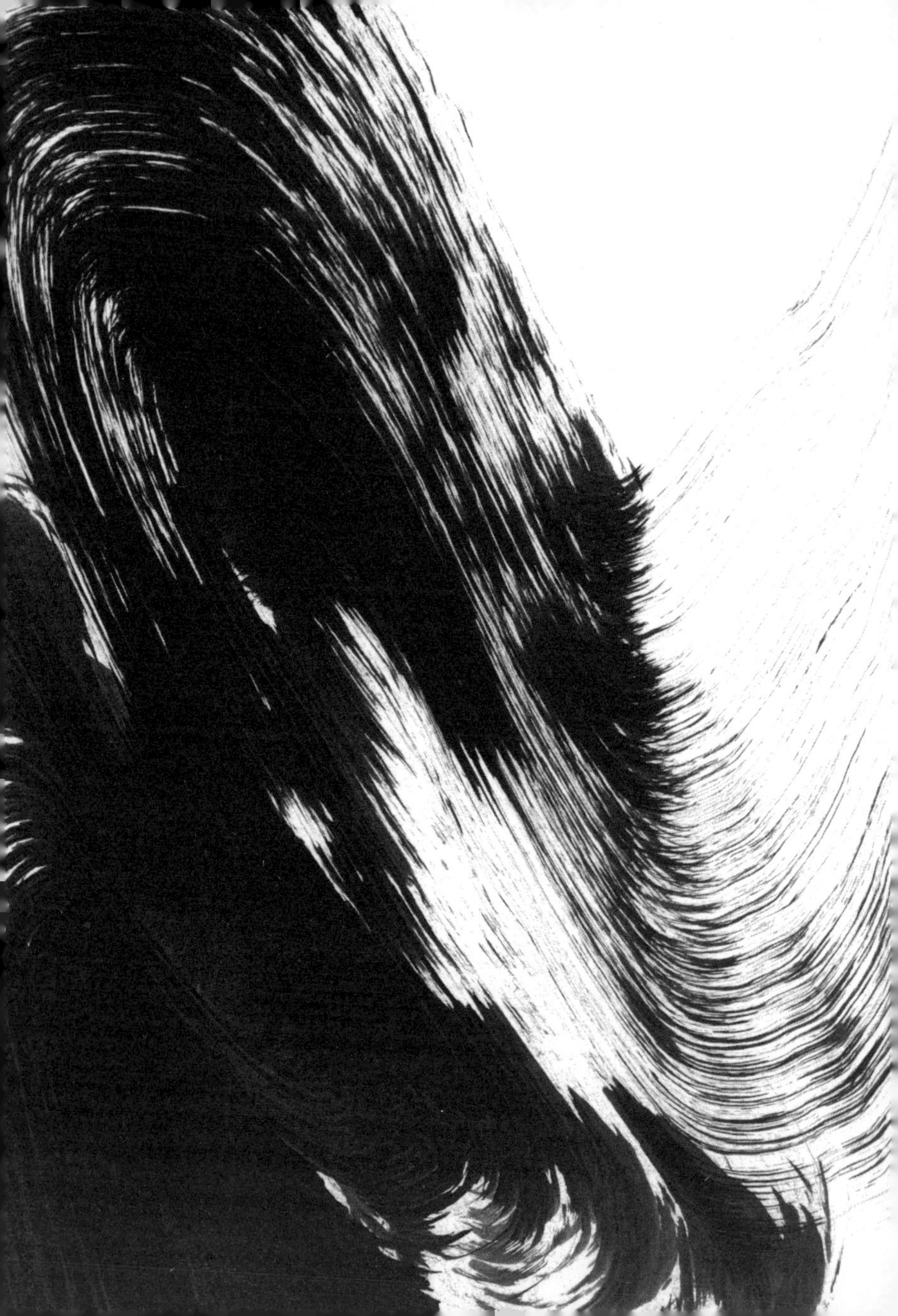

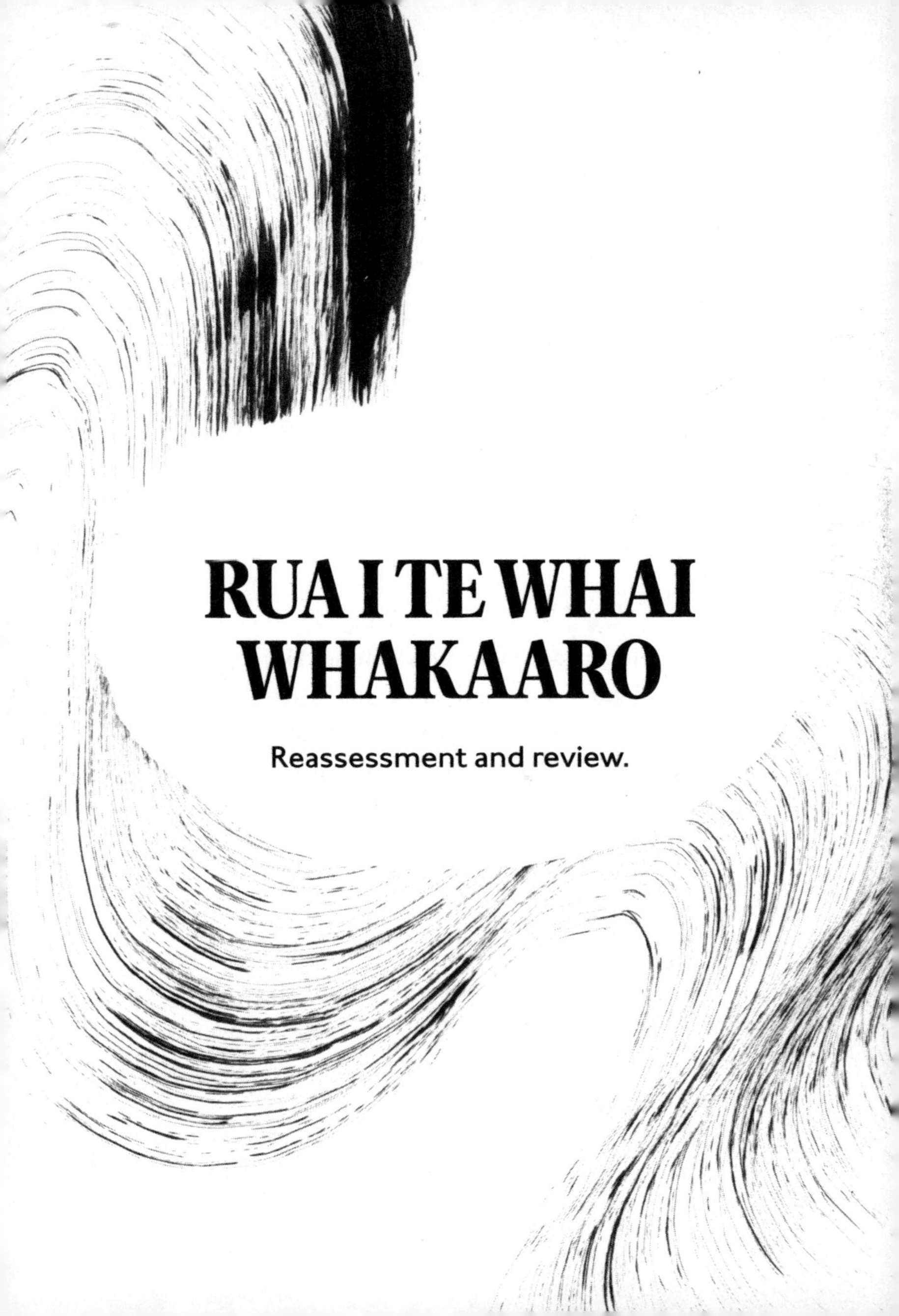

RUA I TE WHAI WHAKAARO

Reassessment and review.

Te Aupōuri.

People who survived by means of smoke and ash.

Leaving our massive lava flow behind, Hinengaro begins to lead us gradually upwards into the cooler air. A steadily flowing stream cuts through the rock, soot remnants peppering the surface. Tiny messages of farewell from Te Whatumanawa. We reach down to stroke the water. The refreshing touch then cools our flushed cheeks. A shift is beginning, our compass curves around, our calves stretching on the upwards incline. We feel a readiness to push on, continuing to process all that Hinengaro is revealing to us.

How fitting to come to a place to review and reflect. The place to mull things over. The silence is deafening. Quite an adjustment after the rumbling pulse of Te Whatumanawa. Our heart rate slows, our lungs soften with gratitude.

We are in a cave of deliberation. Quiet, careful review. Something most of us are unfamiliar with. We are taught that being on the go is how we must live. Filling up any silence with chatter. We learn it is vital to show others how much work we are doing to feel worthy. We wear our economic identity as a badge of honour. We don't get paid to stop and take the time to ponder our life questions, so what is the point, right, where is the value in that? And yet Hinengaro highlights introspection as a crucial need by providing us with this rua i te whai whakaaro. Hinengaro reminds us we must stop here to process our inner pool of resourcefulness.

Deep reflection follows deep emotion. The watery companion to the fire.

For me this is a time when my thoughts return to the story of Whēru. It is said, 'Ko Whēru te rangimārie', 'Whēru, the peacemaker'. As you may know, Whēru was a smart leader who was known as someone who advocated for peace. Sadly for him and his younger brother, Te Ikanui, their sister

Kupe was murdered in an attempt to provoke a war designed to take control of their fertile lands. Revenge was swift: Te Ikanui took out his sister's murderer. But retaliation followed. The murderer's people came back to exact their own payback. Whēru, Te Ikanui and their people were able to withstand their enemies for a while. But they realised this could not go on. They had to carefully review their situation and come up with a feasible strategy for survival.

Picture Whēru, Te Ikanui and their whānau amid the attacks. Finding their own journey into rua i te whai whakaaro, a place of much-needed calm to get their ideas together. An invitation to all of us to settle into reassessment mode. Discovering the deliberation needed to devise the right approach, in the right way. Imagine their wānanga, their debate and consideration of possible scenarios. Eventually they landed on a plan. Collecting dry leaves and wood, they positioned these piles at various points inside their pā. They knew they had to communicate their decisions effectively with their whole community to ensure everyone was on board. Everyone knew their role; everyone knew the timing. At the agreed signal the fires were lit. Smoke billowed out, obscuring the pā. Once this protective cloak of smoke covered the site, the community made their escape by waka and paddled away to safety. The fire continued to rage, towering dark clouds and ash were expelled far into the air. The waters of the Whangapē harbour turned black. Our people's survival was based on the time taken to reassess and formulate a successful plan of escape. The acumen of our wheinga is forever enshrined in the name of our iwi, Te Aupōuri, the people who survived by means of charcoal smoke and inky currents. A very real example of the importance of making time in our very own rua i te whai whakaaro.

How do you find the idea of staying put for a while in your rua i te whai whakaaro? This can feel uncomfortable for many of us at first. We like to be 'doing', not 'being'. You might find yourself asking, what's the point, or you might hear a voice saying, 'I don't have time for this'. It might be difficult to feel the benefits at first. Give Hinengaro a chance to show you the advantages that await you by spending time here. This might be a time to write something down, to document experiences in your hautaka or journal, to consider the phase of Hina, our Māori moon. What are the treasures you find in rua i te whai whakaaro today?

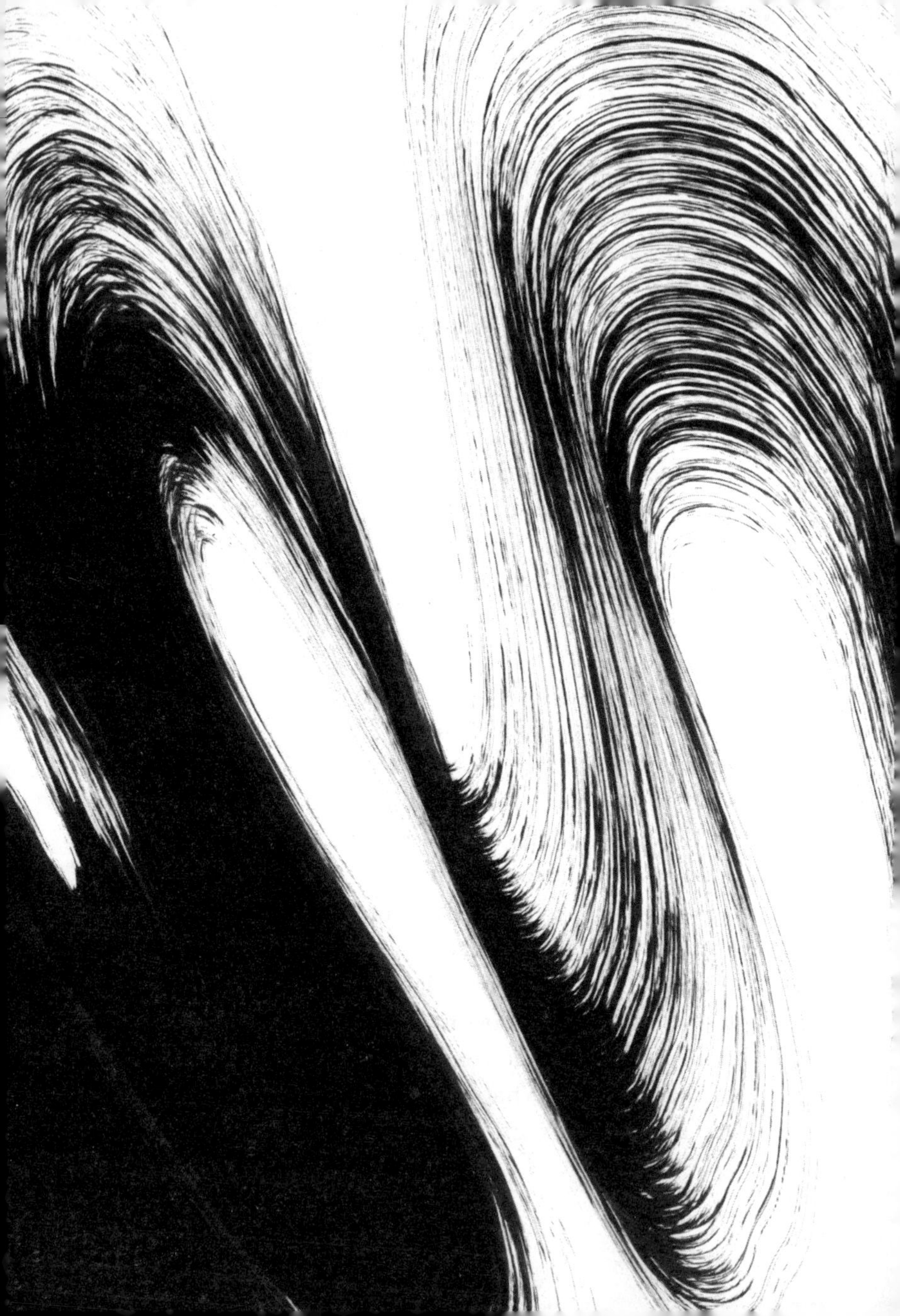

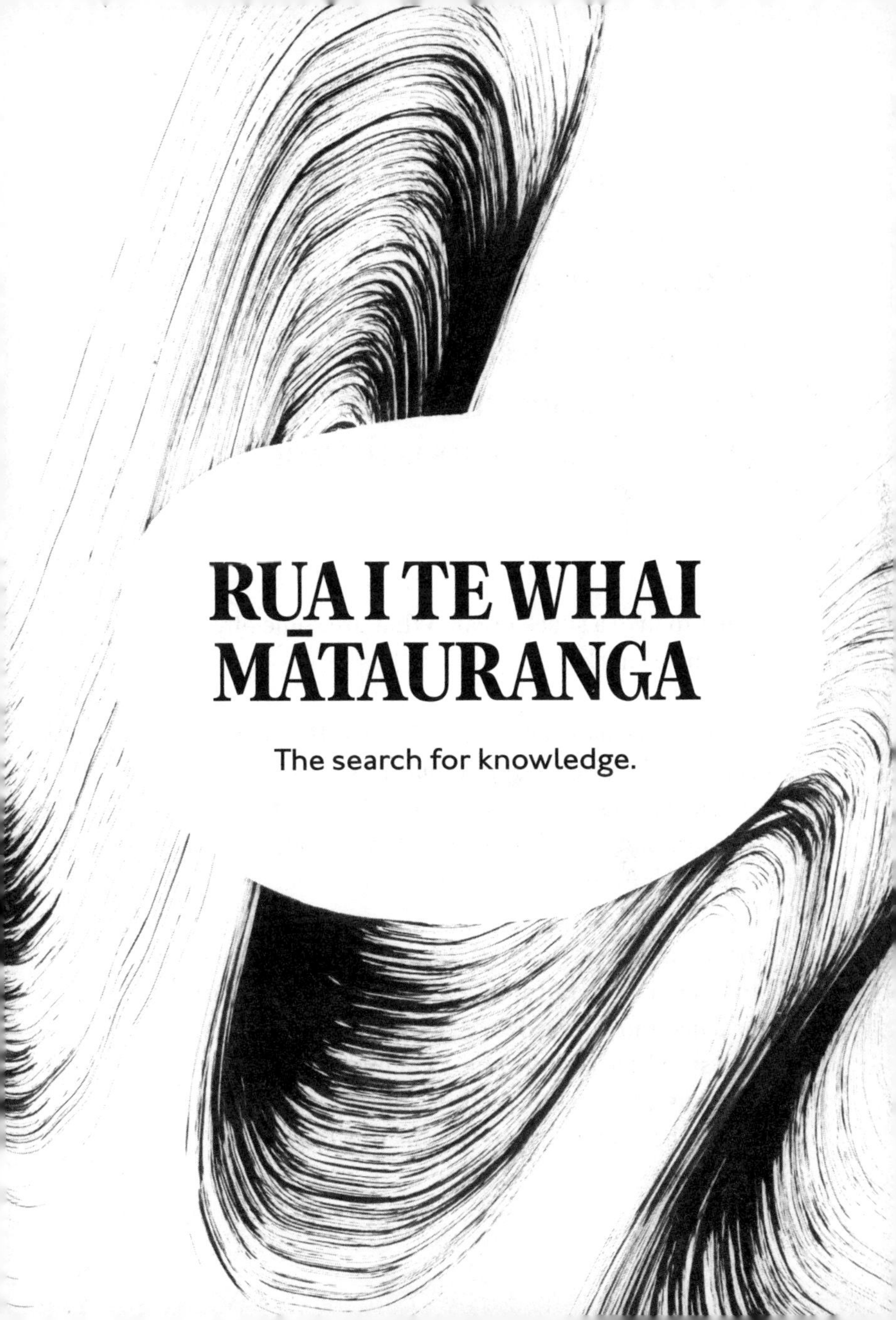

RUA I TE WHAI MĀTAURANGA

The search for knowledge.

Ko te manu e kai ana i te miro nōna te ngahere, ko te manu e kai ana i te mātauranga nōna te ao.

The bird that feeds on the miro berry, theirs is the forest. The bird that feeds on knowledge, theirs is the world.

Time to take a snack break. What are some of your favourite snacks?

We have been on a wild ride through Hinengaro's rua already, discovering so many novel ways to reconsider our lives, inviting freedom of thought and alternative solutions. Kai, food, is our enriching metaphor for our next pit stop.

This famous whakataukī focuses on the contrasting food choices of our manu, our birds. Eating berries or consuming knowledge. This proverbial saying has stood the test of time. One interpretation gives us such a clear picture of the impact on our lives when we continue to consume only what we are most used to, what is easily available, what feeds into our own sense of self protection. Alternatively, we can ingest knowledge, a different and harder-to-find type of nourishment that requires constant effort.

This rua is a place of action. This is not a cave of knowledge itself; it is a place about the pursuit of knowledge.

The light is becoming stronger as we gingerly step upwards into the cave of pearly-white rounded river stones. Smaller white pebbles are arranged across the floor of the cavern and line the walls with mosaic-like precision. Here we meet our quest for knowledge. We totter slightly on the uneven stones. This is not straightforward. Placing our feet more carefully, we begin to chart a way forward, finding our balance. We reach out to touch the smooth skin of these white stones. We sense the responsibility before us.

Our stomachs rumble; we are hungry, eager to begin our quest for knowledge. Our puku, our gut, recognises where we are. Our search for knowledge, for mātauranga, is like digestion; a comprehensive process. When digestion is functioning well, we feel satisfied, satiated. When we have a sore puku, we might feel bloated, bound up and nauseous. Similarly, when we consume different kinds of knowledge it impacts on our feelings. If we are more deliberate about our mind-palates, just like trying out unfamiliar tastes and textures, we can explore knowledge from a range of sources to experience what combinations strangely enhance each other. I imagine Hinengaro relishing the mind-food equivalents of feasting on caramel and sea salt, watermelon and feta cheese, pineapple and coconut, pork and pūhā.

Like our digestive system, the pursuit of knowledge is for life. We process the knowledge we ingest, and we get rid of the waste that doesn't serve us. We are nourished by the goodness that mātauranga provides. This is about lifelong learning. He ara mutunga kore. A path without end. We must take our time with our food too, just like our search for knowledge. Bolting down this kind of food doesn't help. We can only get away with cramming for exams for so long before it takes a toll. A healthy pursuit of knowledge helps us to feel enlightened, to grow in the confidence to make better decisions based on our evolving understanding. In this way we can continue to expand our knowledge, to get better and better at solving our life challenges.

We live in a world of many kinds of knowledge, some of which is designed to be misleading. We must be careful about what we put onto our mind-platter. And to stretch the metaphor a little, we need to consider how the food has been prepared and curated to whet our appetite, or to look appealing, when in fact the food may lack nutrition and be without flavour.

Māori Marsden has written about students of the original whare wānanga, or places of learning. When those in pursuit of mātauranga entered the wharenui they would go to a certain pou, te pou tūārongo, the pillar at the back of the whare. There they would pick up the Hukatai stone, the white stone, and put it in their mouth. After symbolically swallowing the stone, they would replace it. This hands-on experience served as a reminder that the journey of searching for knowledge is an active one to be cherished. Hukatai represents the sea foam, the wake of the waka as it travels across the ocean. The Hukatai signifies the tumultuous path of our never-ending pursuit of knowledge*.

* Marsden, M. & Henare, T.A. (1992). *Kaitiakitanga: A definitive introduction to the holistic world view of the Māori*. Ministry for the Environment.

Don’t get me wrong. I am not suggesting that we are going to put rocks into our mouths. These are metaphorical lessons that help us to activate our own personal way of experiencing knowledge processing and absorption.

What are some aspects of knowledge you feel ready to pursue? Maybe your te reo journey is ready to begin; maybe you have the urge to grow your knowledge of mahinga kai, gardening, so you can provide for your whānau? Or maybe you want to work out how to identify fake news as technology continues to evolve and the accuracy of information becomes harder to authenticate?

I use a pinch of rock salt to remind me about rua i te whai mātauranga, a morsel of edible rock which I can use to add a little extra flavour to my kai. What could you try to remind you of your journey in searching for understanding? How might you create a more deliberate, structured practice of devouring and digesting the knowledge you need?

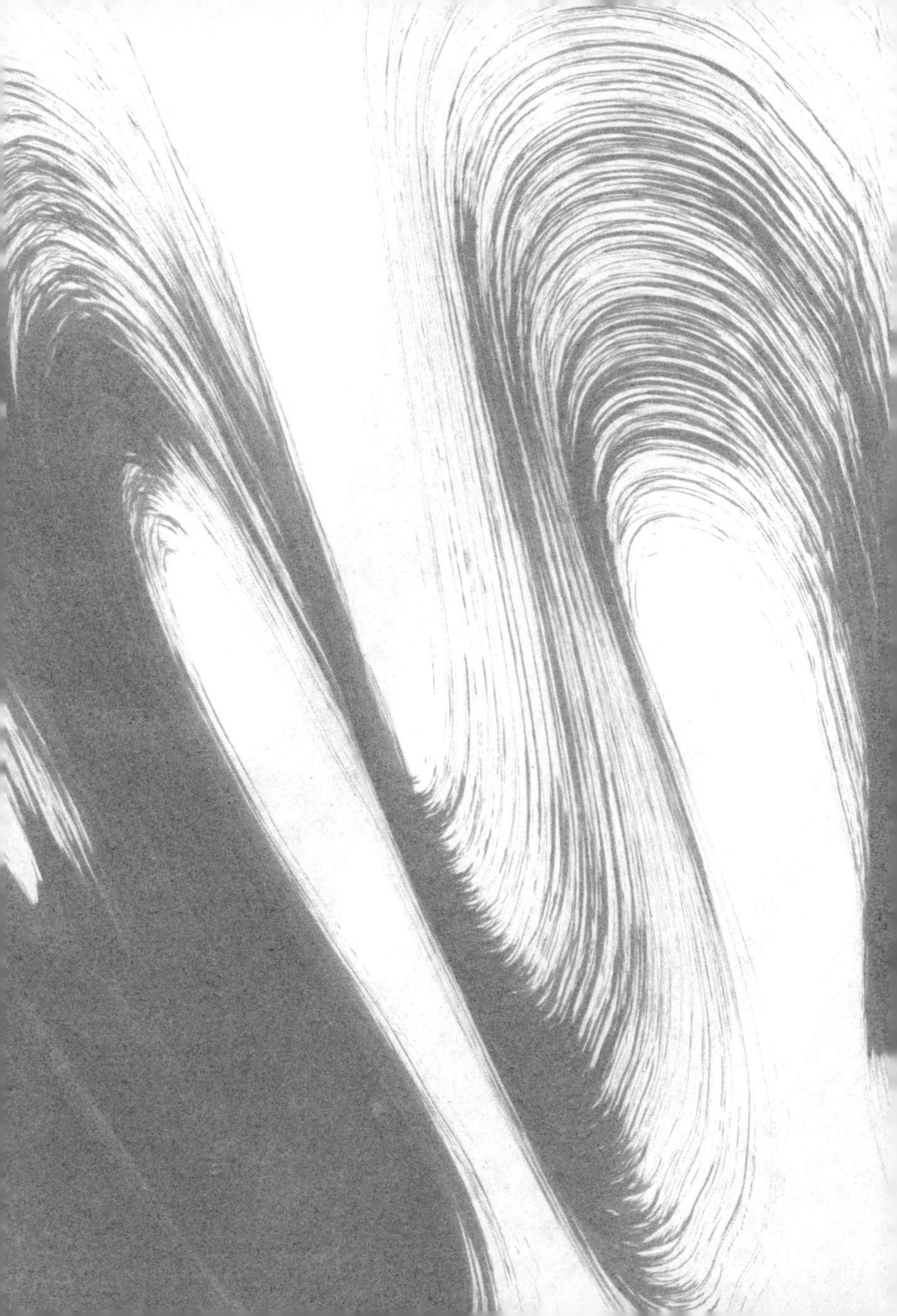

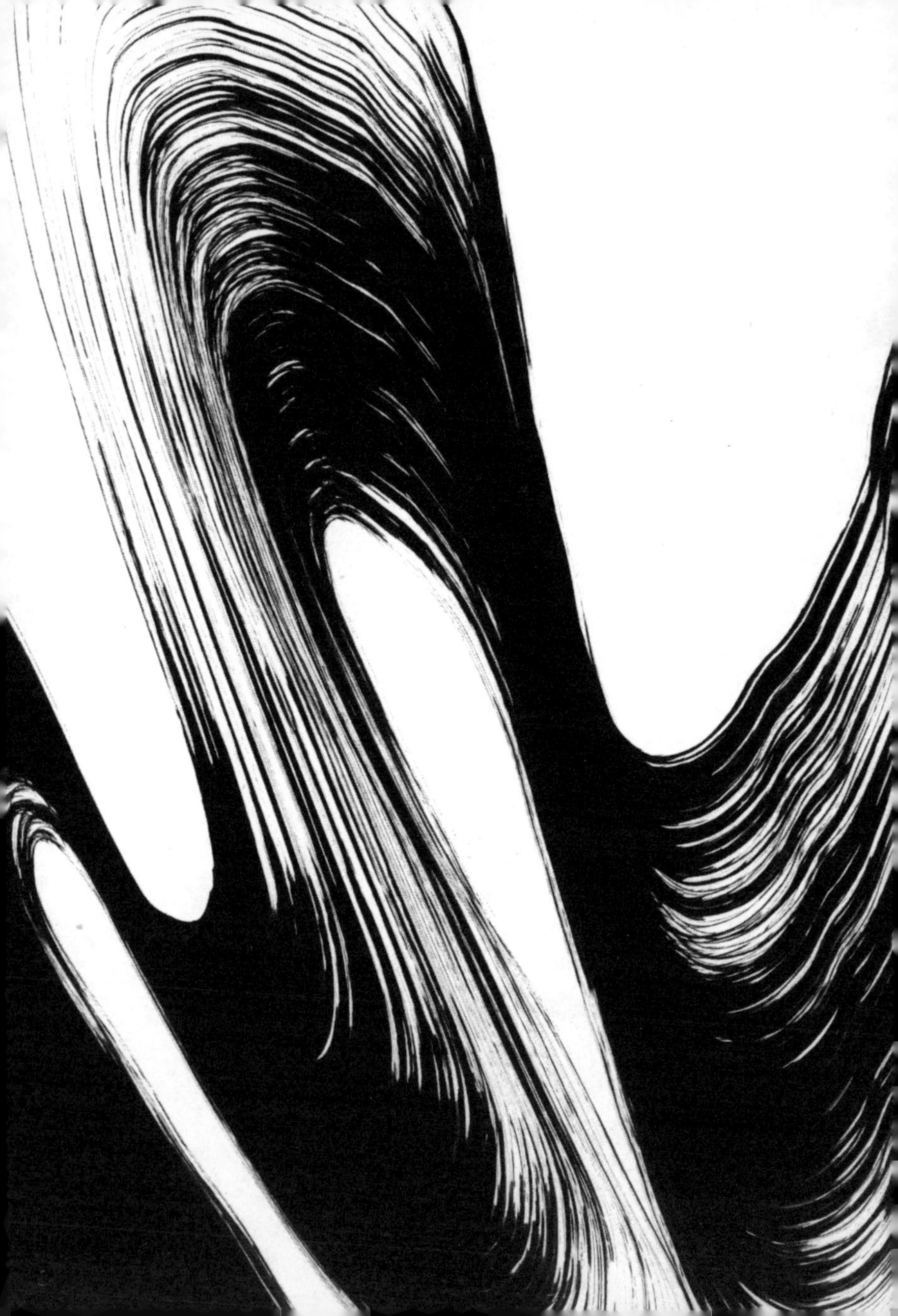

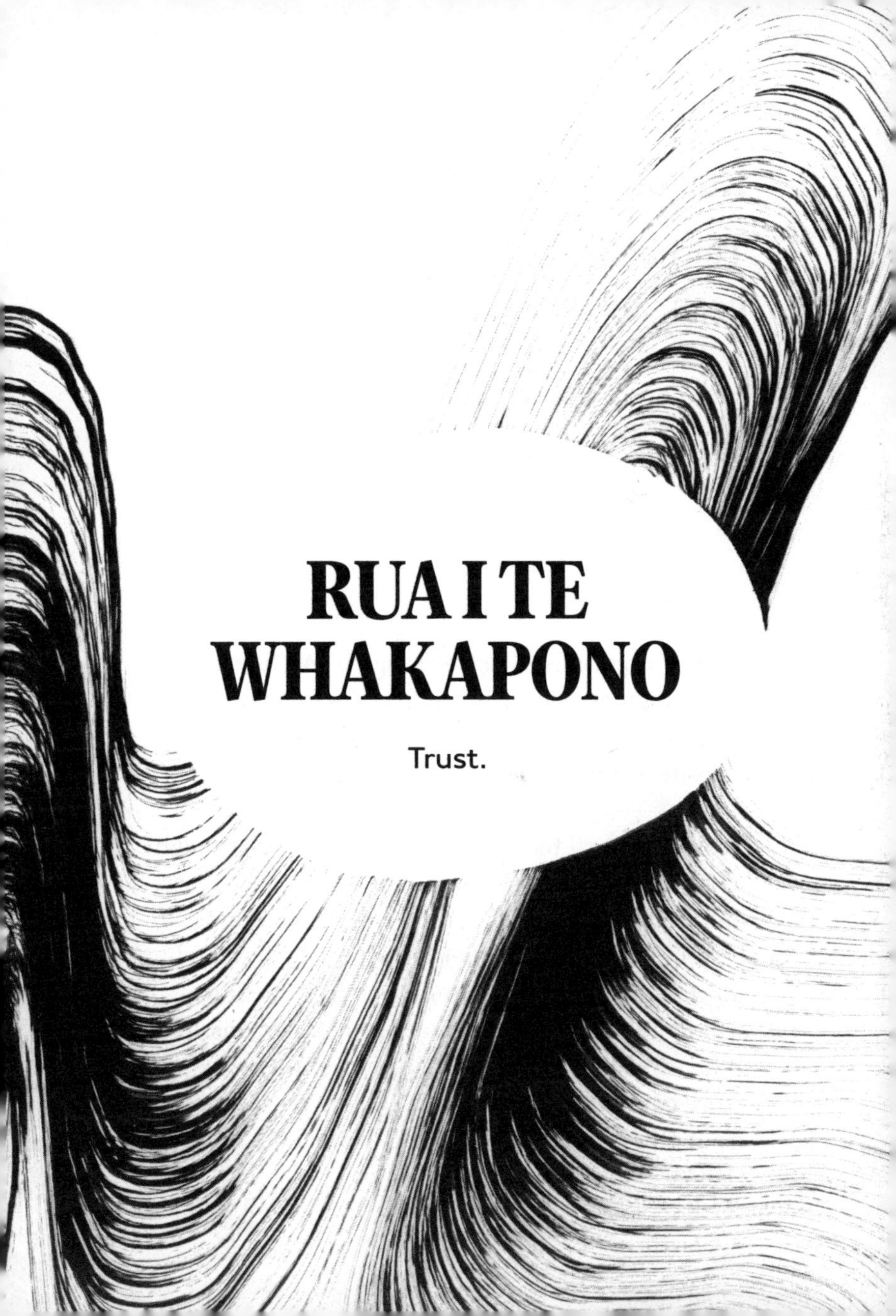

RUA I TE WHAKAPONO

Trust.

Kua takoto te mānuka.

The challenge of trust has been laid down.

Hinengaro brings us upwards again. We turn up a short flight of steps hewn in the rock opening into our rua i te whakapono, our place dedicated to the consideration of trust.

Trust is central to our lives. How we learn through experiences of trust is critical in our earliest years and shapes the rest of our development. Trust can be thought of as the belief that others will reliably do what they say, will honour our relationships, will uphold the reciprocity of our connections. When we have a strong sense of trust we feel more confident in anticipating likely responses from others in the wider world around us. Trust also helps us to stretch our embrace to hold the unexpected, based on our history of trust.

Entering this rua we become acutely aware of our shared intergenerational experiences of trust. We start to become aware of how mistrust works like splintered bark, sharply piercing our emotional skin. These tiny shards that create suspicion and doubt. And it hits home that the spectrum of trust and loss of trust is not solely an individual experience, but a shared one. Without realising it we are walking into our next rua on tiptoe, caution filling us from the legs up. Sensing all those we bring with us to explore our collective history of trust.

Hinengaro has a pōwhiri ready and waiting. We are called forward. Hinengaro herself has laid down a mānuka branch on the ground. Here is her wero, her challenge. Her formal expression of whether this is a trusted encounter, or not. We must consider our back stories of trust with ourselves, with others and with the world.

We stand looking down at the humble mānuka branch. We know what this means. Once the mānuka is picked up, we have indicated our understanding: this is a symbol of reciprocity. A mark of trust in action. Rua i te whakapono floods us with reminders of experiences across our spectrum of trust over the years. Wounds left by betrayal of trust that have added to caution, fear and pain. Parts of ourselves that feel so vulnerable, that have taken years to begin to heal, come into the light. Some are unexpectedly raw. Here we can focus on times where no one took responsibility, no one listened, our need for trust was neglected. Times we trusted, despite the evidence, because we hate to be wrong. Eventually we had to learn the hard way. Our trust was abused. Scanning for threat has taken up so much of our lives.

As a doctor, there is a special kind of trust that we try to establish and maintain with the people we work with. However, many people continue to feel let down by doctors. It is confronting to face the fact that our profession has lost some of the community's trust.

We formally express the trust others place in us during graduation ceremonies via oaths, many of which stem from the famous Hippocratic oath. I was honoured to represent our graduating medical class by reading our oath in our reo rangatira, our Māori language. Kaumātua Pineaha Murray and Selwyn Muru put the ceremonial cloak from Merimeri Penfold around my shoulders. A solemn, unforgettable moment.

Our oath began like this: 'Ka ōati pono ahau ki te whai i runga i te ngākau atawhai, te kaupapa hauora, me ngā mea e tika ana mō te tohunga whakaora.' 'I promise to be caring in seeking the aspects of hauora, being truthful, ethical and accurate as a specialist working in supporting restoration of health and wellbeing.'

One particular phrase that continues to shine out is this: 'Me taku whakaae ki te pīkau pono i aku mahi me te tuku māramatanga ki ērā atu, hei tohu māharatanga ki ōku kaiwhakaako . . .' 'And my promise is to carry sincerity in my work and share understanding with others as a way of honouring those who have taught me . . .'

Our oath continues to travel with me as new challenges have emerged in health systems, impacting patients, their whānau, communities and our workforce. Pandemics leading to massive shifts in how we deliver safe and compassionate care. Workforce shortages and burnout becoming our shared reality. Pressures from climate emergencies meaning doctors have not been able to reach certain areas. Wars limiting or preventing access to the people who need us the most. For displaced peoples from different cultures, we struggle to build trust. Language and cultural differences make deeply trusting bonds hard to establish and maintain.

No matter what our roles in life, no matter our generational age and stage, our shared experiences of trust, our belief in the availability of trust is profoundly shaken. The future of trust is in jeopardy. The hidden agendas, the repeated broken promises, the half-truths. The deliberate and predatory misinformation now so common in our world. Trusting can feel so naive. Our experiences of trust feel downtrodden.

Looking down at the branch, we can see the flecks of bark ready to draw blood if we pick it up in the wrong way. There is a long exhalation, our unconscious breath releases our fears and we reach down. Picking up the mānuka branch firmly, trusting ourselves and the insight Hinengaro has given to us. There is such clarity of reciprocity. Instilling trust into our connections with others and the world around us. We begin to feel re-energised.

Hinengaro provides rua i te whakapono for us to commit to learning to trust. Holding this mānuka branch, holding our own personal challenge, we are expanding our sense of trust, at our own pace, in our own way.

Rua i te whakapono is our place to return to this essential aspect of our lives and of our wellbeing. Here we take time and energy to explore this basic aspect of our lives. What does picking up the mānuka branch of trust mean to you? How can you take time here to reflect on the evolving relationship you and yours have with trust? Consider our roles in healing trust patterns within our whānau, our extended families and our communities. How can we pass on experiences of trust to our babies, our tamariki mokopuna, our future generations?

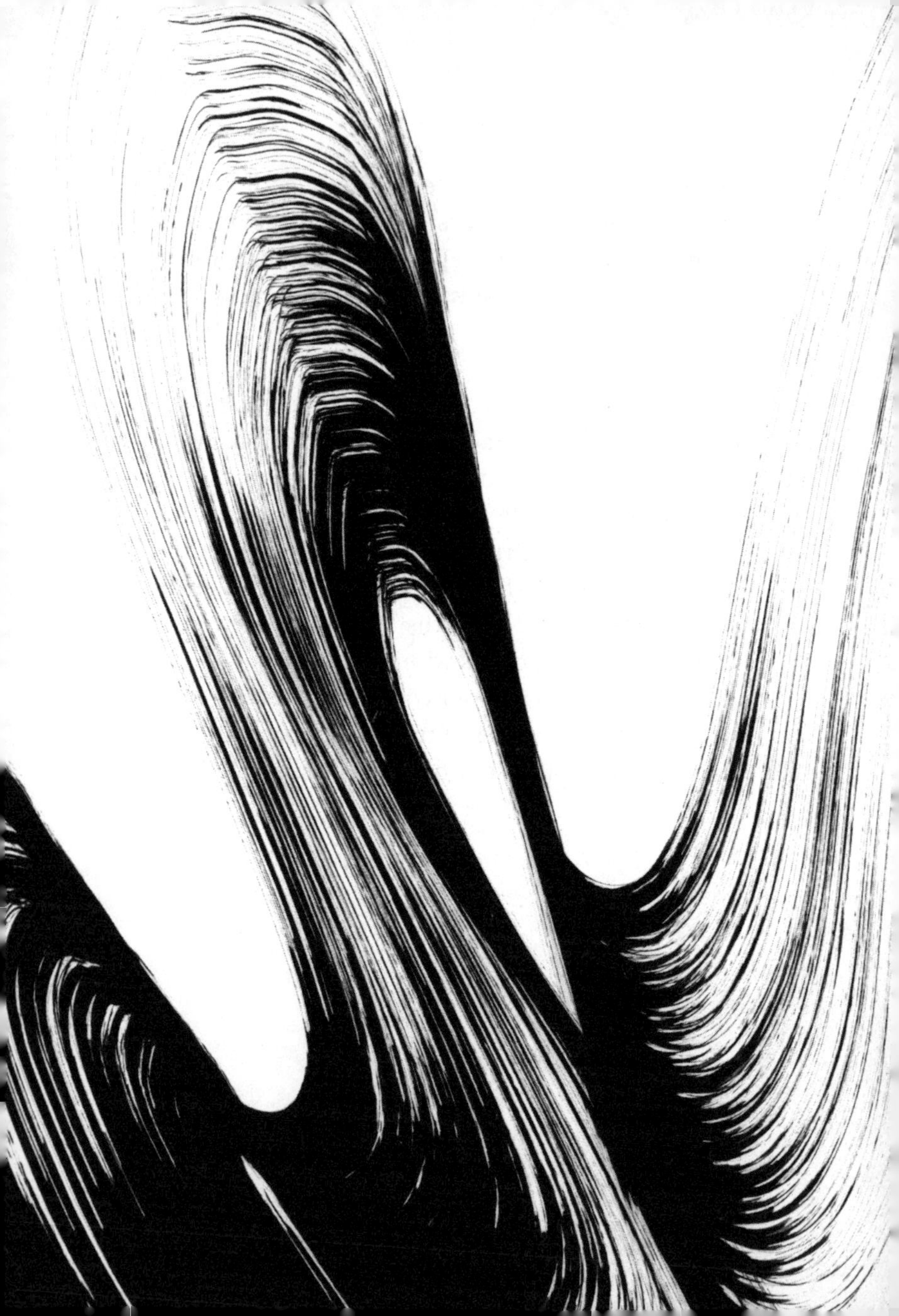

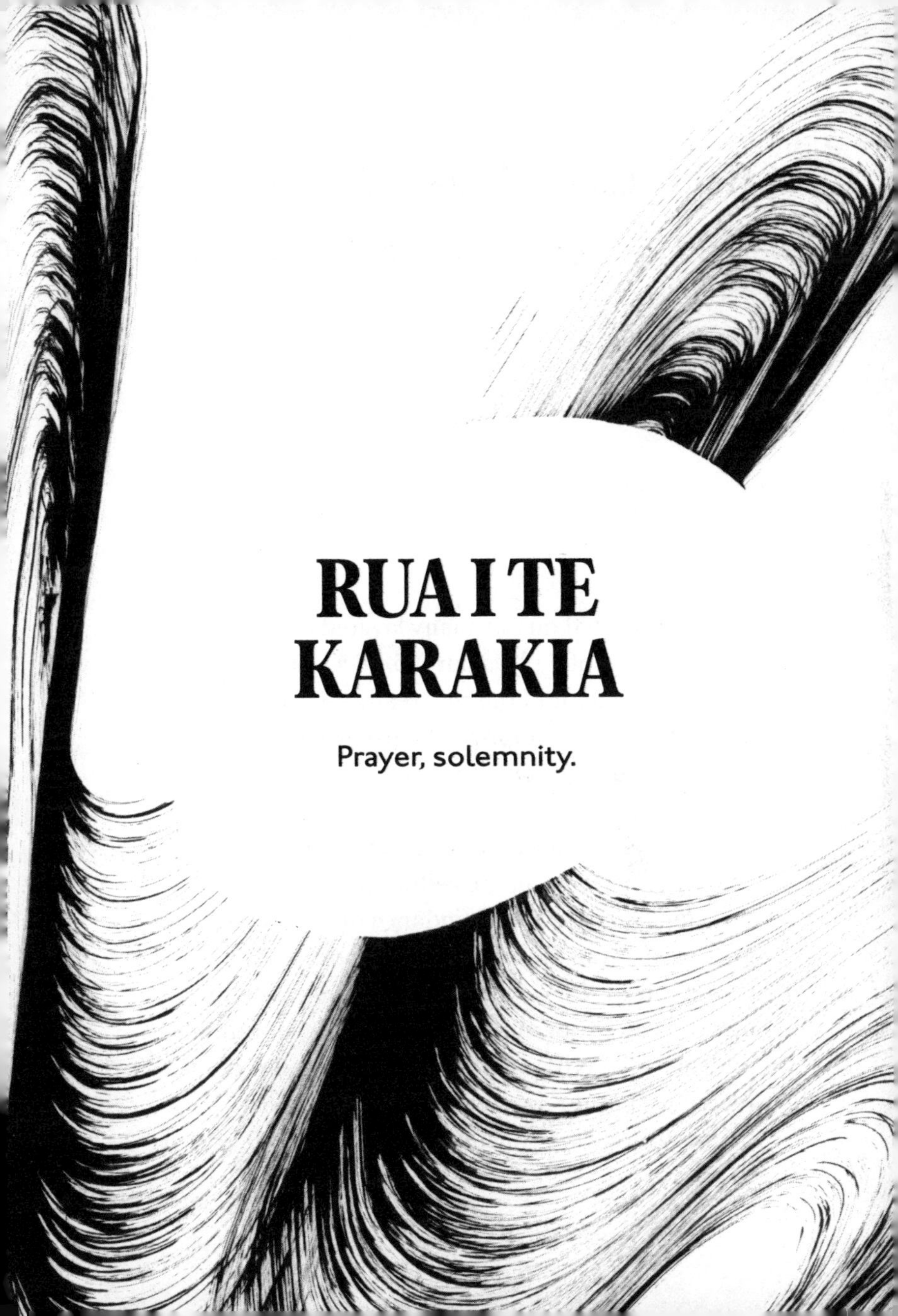

RUA I TE KARAKIA

Prayer, solemnity.

Hokianga whakapau karakia.

Hokianga that exhausts incantation.

Having reflected on our many layered experiences of trust, we gently place our mānuka branch back down on the floor of the rua, ready for our return. We carry our own imprint of trust as Hinengaro guides us onwards and upwards.

Just a few steps away we find ourselves in a vast, expansive cave, the ceiling reaching up to dizzying heights. The abundance of Hinengaro's gifts renews our wellspring of purpose and resourcefulness. We have been moving steadily upwards after our emergence from the emotional inferno of Te Whatumanawa, our reminder of reassessment for survival in whai whakaaro, the mind-food we consume in rua i te whai mātauranga, and lessons about trust are still fresh from rua i te whakapono. Now we encounter rua i te karakia. The atmosphere resonates with the echoes of incantation and chants, prayers and invocation.

We know that our wheinga had their own practices of reciting prayers for all aspects of daily life. Prayers to be conducted upon waking and at the setting of the sun. Prayers for safety and protection in every aspect of birth and death. Prayers for the recognition of connection in every facet of how and why we move in the world.

In Te Tai Tokerau, we have a famous reminder of the power of karakia in the story of Nukutawhiti and Ruanui. These men settled in the harbour of Hokianga: Nukutawhiti to the north, and Ruanui in the south. Each wanted to build their own whare wānanga, place of learning. Establishing their own institutions would ensure the passing on of knowledge, essential to the wellbeing and flourishing of the people.

Nukutawhiti wanted both whare wānanga to be opened ceremonially at the same time. But Ruanui finished early and was keen to open his centre first. Nukutawhiti was annoyed. He was the elder relation, so his wishes needed to be given due respect and priority. Ruanui seemingly ignored tikanga and began his karakia. He used the power of his incantations to invite a whale to come in to shore near his new complex. Perhaps he was trying to demonstrate his own prowess with the power of his chants. Nukutawhiti was not happy about this, so he began his own recitation of karakia, pulling the whale to the northern side. This karakia battle continued until both had exhausted their vocabulary of chants. I imagine them both completely spent, spiritually, mentally and physically. Not to mention how the whale felt.

A few years ago, I was asked to write a karakia. It was a wonderful and daunting challenge. I took time to journey through ngā rua a Hinengaro preparing myself, paying attention to the lessons Hinengaro provided for me. And I was careful to seek the blessings from one of our revered kaumātua for this, 'He karakia ki a Papatūānuku', prayer for Mother Earth.

E Whae, e Papa e hora nei

Mother, Papatūānuku, your great
expanse here before us

te whaea o te tangata

the mother of people

whakarongo mai rā

hear us

ki te ruahine

the female leaders

ki te pukenga

the uprising

ki tō whakahina

your grey-haired

ko Hina i te pō

acknowledging Hina at night

ko Hina i te ao

Hina during the day

ki Hina āmio ki runga

Hina orbiting above

ko Hina whakarite tai

Hina who puts the tides in order

kia puta ko tai tamatāne

bringing forth the oceans of the West Coast

ko tai tamawāhine
the oceans of the East Coast

ko te Tai o Rehua e . . . i.
the oceans of the North.

Rāhiritia atu rā te ūkaipō
Greeting the home sanctuary you provide

kua hua ko te hiringa
the fruits of perseverance

te hiringa tapu
the sacred vitality

te hiringa ā Nuku
the inspiration from you, our source

te wahine pū o te ao
female power of the world

hei ora mō te ao
providing life to benefit the world

hei mana mō te ao
with authority concerning the world

tū i te ao
remaining steadfastly in the world

ko te tū nui

the great stance

ko te tū roa

the long established

ko te tū tē ū

unyielding

ko te tū tē ea

without end

ko te tūrangawaewae

the place to stand

ko te tū oranga tonutanga

the source of health and wellbeing

hui e . . .

together

Tāiki e.*

bound together for ever.

* Elder, H. (2023). He karakia ki a Papatūānuku. In W. Ihimaera. & M. Elvy (eds.), *Whakaruru-taha. A Kind of Shelter. An anthology of new writing for a changed world* (p. 9). Massey University Press.

~

There are many reminders here about the power of karakia as we stand reverently in this vast cave. Here we are immersed in the sacred power of ancient words radiating out into Papatūānuku herself, and from her out into the universe. Some of us face in a specific direction, some close our eyes. For some of us there is an order of acknowledgement and recognition of deities. You might feel yourself beginning to pray. Lips moving silently perhaps. Your own karakia rising with exactly what you need to communicate in this moment. The mesmeric pulse of prayer resonating in the vast chamber of the cave. The power of this sacred sound.

How do we strengthen our innate sense of prayer? Our grave solemnity is a source of such solace. What can we pray for, and how? We might find it easiest to start with our loved ones, their health and long lives. The restoration of our planet, the rediscovery of community and how intimately connected we all are might follow. Allowing our own confidence to build, tuning in to hearing our voices, out loud in prayer. This can feel quite strange at first. Hinengaro reminds us that these sacred practices are not luxuries, they are necessities for our wellbeing. Our karakia include our own awe and reverence for Papatūānuku, our Mother Earth, all her offspring, and our renewed commitment to serve her and future generations.

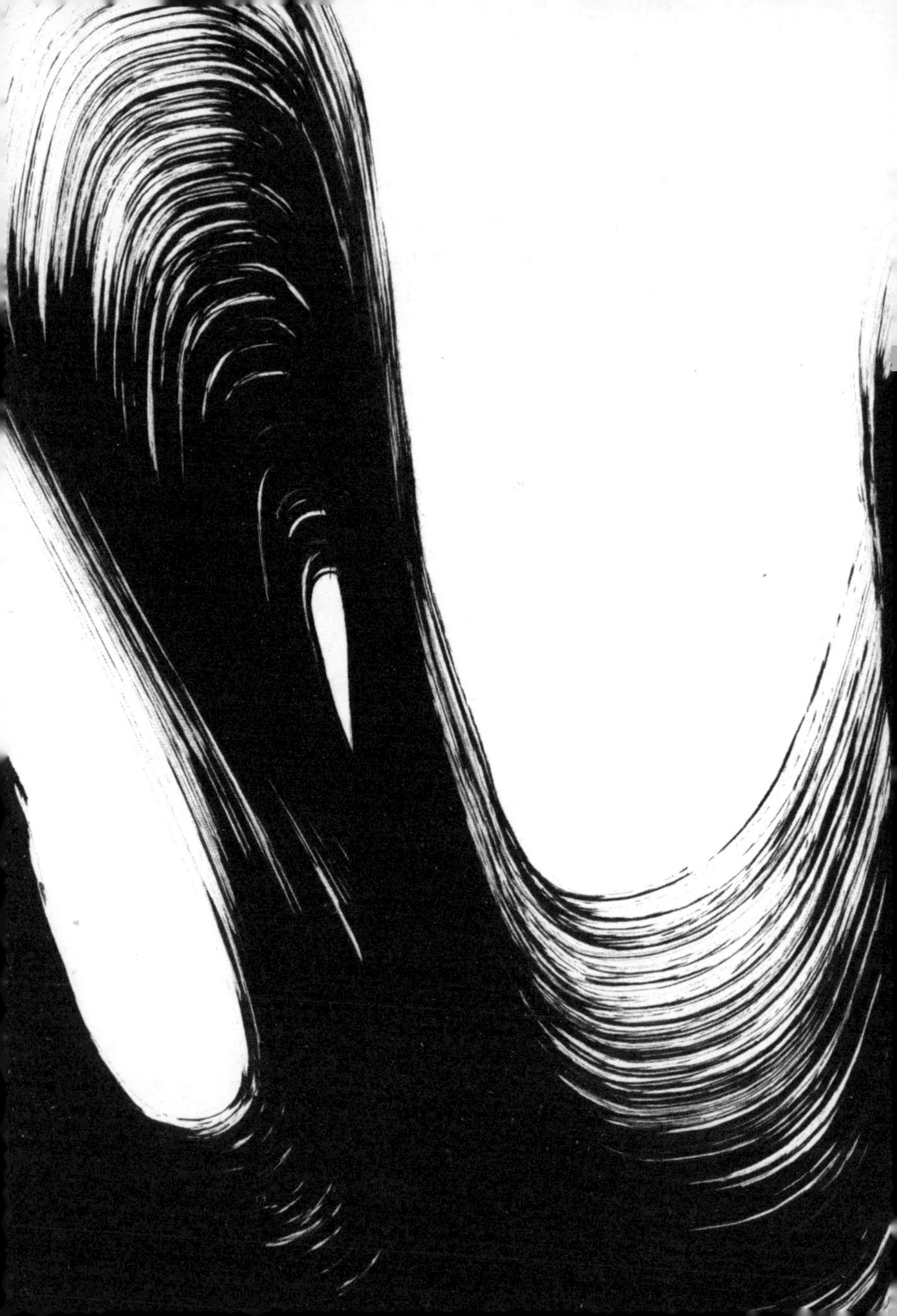

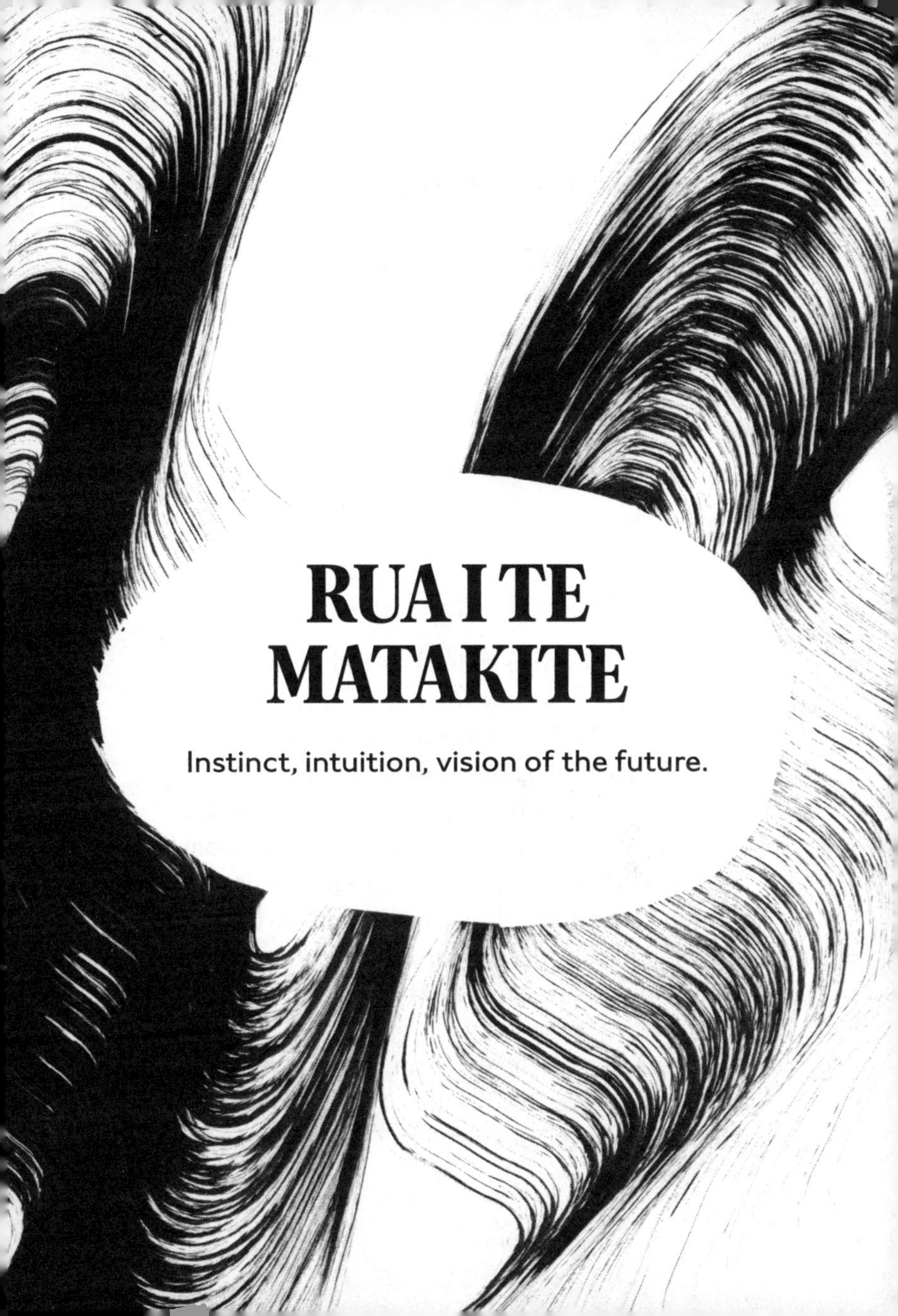

RUA I TE MATAKITE

Instinct, intuition, vision of the future.

Te mātiro whakamua.

Vision beyond the horizon.

Hinengaro continues to lead us on her carefully curated caving journey. We are already feeling the relief of shedding old ways of thinking about thinking. Past their use-by date patterns that never felt like they belonged, like someone else's ill-fitting clothes. Cultural hand-me-downs from another place with another language. We have just felt the intimate impact of karakia, with one example of solemn surrender in homage to Papatūānuku, our earth mother.

Our immersion in the power of prayer is still fresh as we move steadily upwards, entering the realm of intuition and instinct. These rocks feel familiar. Déjà vu. Is this a place from childhood or a recurrent dream? A carved entrance greets us with layer upon layer of ridges in the rocks, inviting the light touch of our fingers. We touch millennia, like the rings of an ancient tree, like the layers on the lip of our treasured shells, collected wandering along the sands where the harakeke once grew. Reminders of the remnants of these creatures' homes, their tiny spacecraft providing their own meditation in our hands. This portal pulls us in, foretelling visions of the future.

The concept of matakite has many layers. It can refer to everyday experiences when we have a strange, knowing feeling. Maybe something doesn't feel quite right; intuition in the pit of our gut. Or we feel a sense of clarity that we are on exactly the right path. No such thing as coincidence. When life events fall into place with ease, somehow there is an alignment. This can be what we call matakite.

Have you ever had one of those moments where you felt all the strands of your life had come together? When you knew you were exactly where you were meant to be, doing exactly what you were destined to do? Time standing completely still.

You could see and feel all the experiences that had brought you to that precise moment. Finally everything made sense.

I want to tell you about one of those moments in my life, where I had such a strong sense of this continuum that we are all part of, whether we like it or not. Being part of the legacy of previous generations who have led the way, and forming the legacy for those who will continue the journey. That infinite connection that curves around us and across time, that we get glimpses of in those extraordinary moments of clarity.

Let me take you to that moment. I am standing in the gateway of an urban marae in West Auckland, the waharoa of Hoani Waititi marae. I am waiting for the karanga that will draw our group forward and which I will respond to across the ātea, the wide space in front of the wharenui. A group of kaumātua and neuroscientists are the manuhiri, the guests. I am suddenly aware of all the stories and all the people that have brought me to this precise moment in time. A deep, gut-level sense of purpose and of vision. Stories that flash through my mind in those milliseconds.

My mother's presence is so clear. Even though she passed away more than 30 years ago from breast cancer, when I was pregnant with my son, today she is right by my side.

My mother saw beyond her own life in ways I did not realise back then. Her legacy was to open my eyes to the possibility of becoming a doctor. From Hinengaro's rua i te matakite an unexpected vision of myself as a doctor of the future crept in. Our mum's dying wish was to gift her body to the medical school, a big deal for a Māori woman and for us, her whānau. And so my mother's life and death led me to medical training. She passed on to me a place in Te Waka Kuaka, the flock of godwits, as her tamariki. Mum showed me how to take my place flying through the migrations of specialist training and daily work, doctoral and postdoctoral research, all of which led me here, to this moment at the waharoa. To this sacred sandbank where kuaka come to settle safely, before the next migration.

This journey did not feel like a straight line. Like our takarangi — our double spiral Māori code, signifying the negative and positive spaces, back through time to our origins — Hinengaro's coiled pathway was the map I followed. Looking back I can see these twists and turns, diving down and then being lifted up on circling currents of air, leading this kuaka to where I needed to be.

Matakite can also mean second sight. The ability to predict events, to have communication with our wheinga. People with these abilities often come from lines of whakapapa where these gifts travel within the whānau. Sometimes people who might be thought of as having a mental illness actually have matakite. So it is vital to have senior cultural supports present to ensure these situations are appropriately identified and that culturally meaningful assistance is put in place.

What aspects of instinct do you recognise and act on? Or do you tend to choose to ignore your intuition and then regret that later on? Do you have some clear recollections of when seemingly disparate aspects of life combined, like the formation of a flock of birds heading in one direction? Or do you feel like part of an endless murmuration where the flock is weaving and turning, in what feels like an erratic and pointless way?

Here is a necessary place Hinengaro has prepared to give us the time and space to explore the importance of matakite. Sometimes these feelings and sensations might be frowned on or dismissed. But just because we cannot yet identify the cause, or how to measure such experiences, does not make them invalid.

I have learned to listen carefully to our whānau and take their insights and hunches seriously. How can we learn to respect and strengthen these aspects of intuition? Rua i te matakite reminds us that our intuitive skills give us data about being connected. Our matakite has its own karanga across the ātea of our lives. Here we can begin to appreciate why Hinengaro makes this a priority.

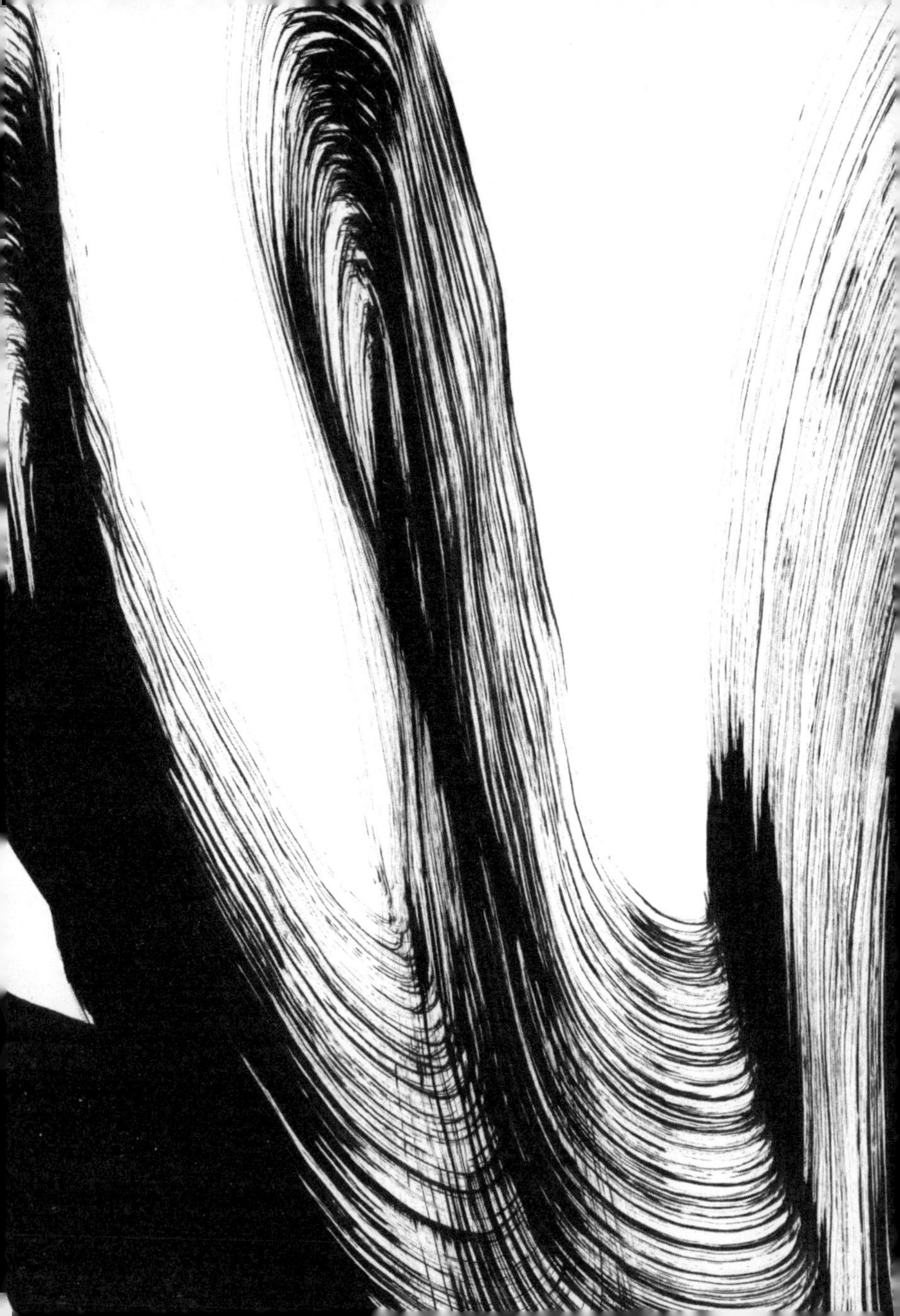

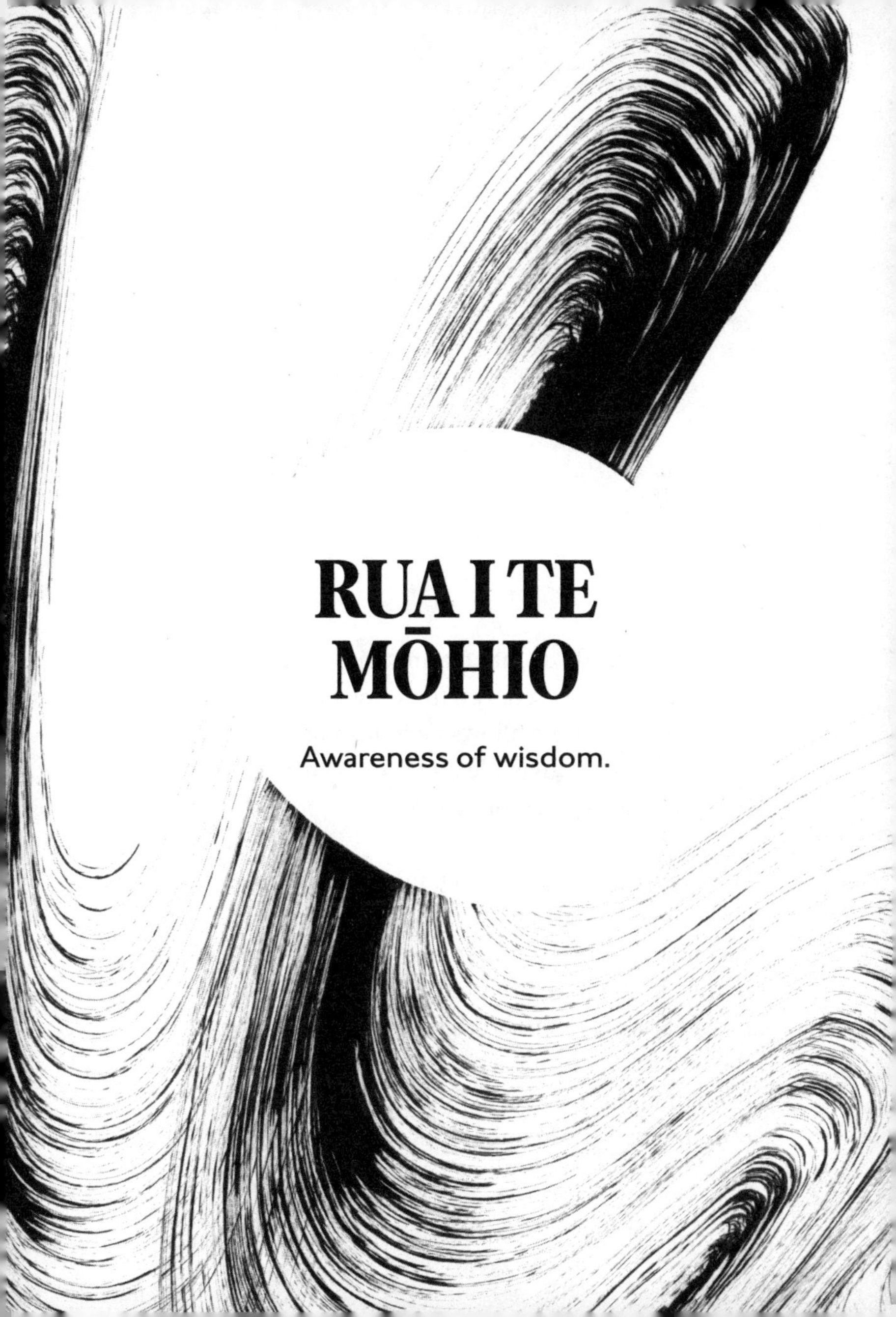

RUA I TE MŌHIO

Awareness of wisdom.

Rehutai.

The red stone.

Hinengaro leads us into a crimson cave. A profoundly settled energy surrounds us. The soft velvety atmosphere allows us to lean on the thick air and feel that invisible embrace. The weighted-blanket effect of wisdom descends.

We have been experiencing our most intuitive selves and now we curve into a vast plush cave where, curiously, there is a fine mist of sea spray hanging in the air. A gentle breeze is blowing, wafting these tiny pearls of water across the cave. We can smell the ocean. It is as if we are witnessing the red dawn from onboard a waka, sailing beyond the horizon into the future. Morning's rosy glow signals our passage through the waves. Here in our cave, beams of light glance through cracks in the roof. Rainbows hang suspended, arching across our path. Colours cling onto the air in a mirage.

Hinengaro casts our thoughts back to rua i te mātauranga where we ceremonially swallowed Hukatai, the white stone. We felt the rush of information available to us in those moments. Much to digest. Since then, we have continued through Hinengaro's rua of whakapono, trust and belief, karakia, prayer, and matakite, via the multi-layered portal of our visionary natures — all elements Hinengaro deems necessary for the transition from the search for knowledge to an awareness of wisdom. She has prepared the way.

Hinengaro gives us opportunities to enhance our own true core, where knowledge is transformed into wisdom. Where we can face the big questions in life. This is also a spiritual experience where the puzzles, contradictions and tensions in our lives can begin to feel some sense of resolution. It might feel like wisdom is a long way off in this moment. And yet here is a place to visit that possibility, the beginning of that inkling.

Wisdom is a concept that we have been taught to feel is something reserved for people other than ourselves. We get the idea that wisdom is reserved for the very old, those who have lived through many hardships. Only they have the ability to gracefully assess a situation, weighing up all the elements in order to make quality decisions. And we might be fortunate enough to have examples in our lives that show this can be true.

Hinengaro shows us a broader view. She brings us here to remind us wisdom is something we are all developing throughout our lives. Wisdom can be thought of as happening via compression. Like the rocks surrounding us, we are changing under pressure all this time. That is how we can begin to form our own nuggets of wisdom. A certain alchemy is made possible when we survive pain and suffering, and remind ourselves there are lessons on the way. Often those lessons are hard to see through the tears, fear, rage and searing grief. The first time our hearts are shattered, the first time we are betrayed, lied to, face disease and the death of loved ones, we find ourselves without any reference points. The unspeakable shock and loss feels insurmountable. We don't know where to turn.

Slowly, like ancient rocks, we find ways to hold on. Like the almost imperceptible growth of helictite forms, taking a hundred years to grow one centimetre, we try to find the lesson and learn something from it. So the next time we are hurt we have something to compare this to.

Over and over again life presents tragedy. Hinengaro shows us this is how we begin to build and shape what will one day become wisdom.

A heaped mound of vermilion pebbles, kōwhatu, emerges from the shimmering rainbows floating in the air. The image is so exquisitely beautiful. Tears begin to fall down our cheeks. We feel the reverence in placing one of these vermilion stones gently on the tongue. Closing our mouths we imagine swallowing this talisman of wisdom.

Whether it feels like the first or the one-thousandth dose of wisdom, we accept our part in finding wisdom in our lives.

What enigmas are you feeling overwhelmed by right now? How could you take a small step towards shaping the information you have into a perspective that gives you a glimpse of some element of wisdom?

Perhaps it is about stepping back from all the facts and taking a broader view. I sometimes imagine what the problem might look like if I were on a waka on the ocean, or from a whetū, a star, in outer space.

When we take the scarlet kōwhatu into our mouths, Rehutai asks us, 'what would our ancestors say?' How might they formulate these facts, this data? The old people might say something seemingly tangential. Or they might be blunt. We can imagine they would reference an observation from nature, tested over time in their own ways, the lessons they discovered to ensure the people flourished. We can follow their lead and do something along the same lines. Creating a whakatauākī, a proverb, to synthesise all the flotsam and jetsam of knowledge accumulated in our lives can help. I was inspired to write such a whakatauākī by my frustration in talking to people from some other cultures about the challenges we face in te ao Māori, the Māori world. Their response was often, 'really?', said in an incredulous tone as if to say, 'that can't be true, I don't believe you, you are wrong'. I sat with my irritation and sense of being disrespected and disbelieved. Writing this whakatauākī helped me to articulate what I was feeling and give feedback in a way that I felt was constructive: 'Horekau a Tātarāmoa e takahia ana te mana e Kōhi'. 'The mana of the tātarāmoa (bush lawyer) can never be surmounted by the gorse bush'. Both the gorse and the tātarāmoa are plants that have thorns. Gorse comes from outside of Aotearoa and is smaller. Tātarāmoa turuhunga, as it is also known, is indigenous, and provides abundant fruit, sustaining birds and people. It can be used as an anxiolytic — a remedy for anxiety — and an aid for sleep. It is a shrub that is referenced in oratory and texts, opening up the world to its own wisdom. Plus, it has sharp curved talons which hook onto your clothes, refusing to let go. Tātarāmoa is not to be messed with. Composing this whakatauākī helped me to create a compact yet measured response, holding so many cultural layers. And I felt much better.

How could writing a whakatauākī shift your mind-currents towards wisdom? Turn the rudder of Hinengaro's wisdom waka towards the blushing face of dawn. Witness the sea-spray rainbow and find the course that wisdom has for you.

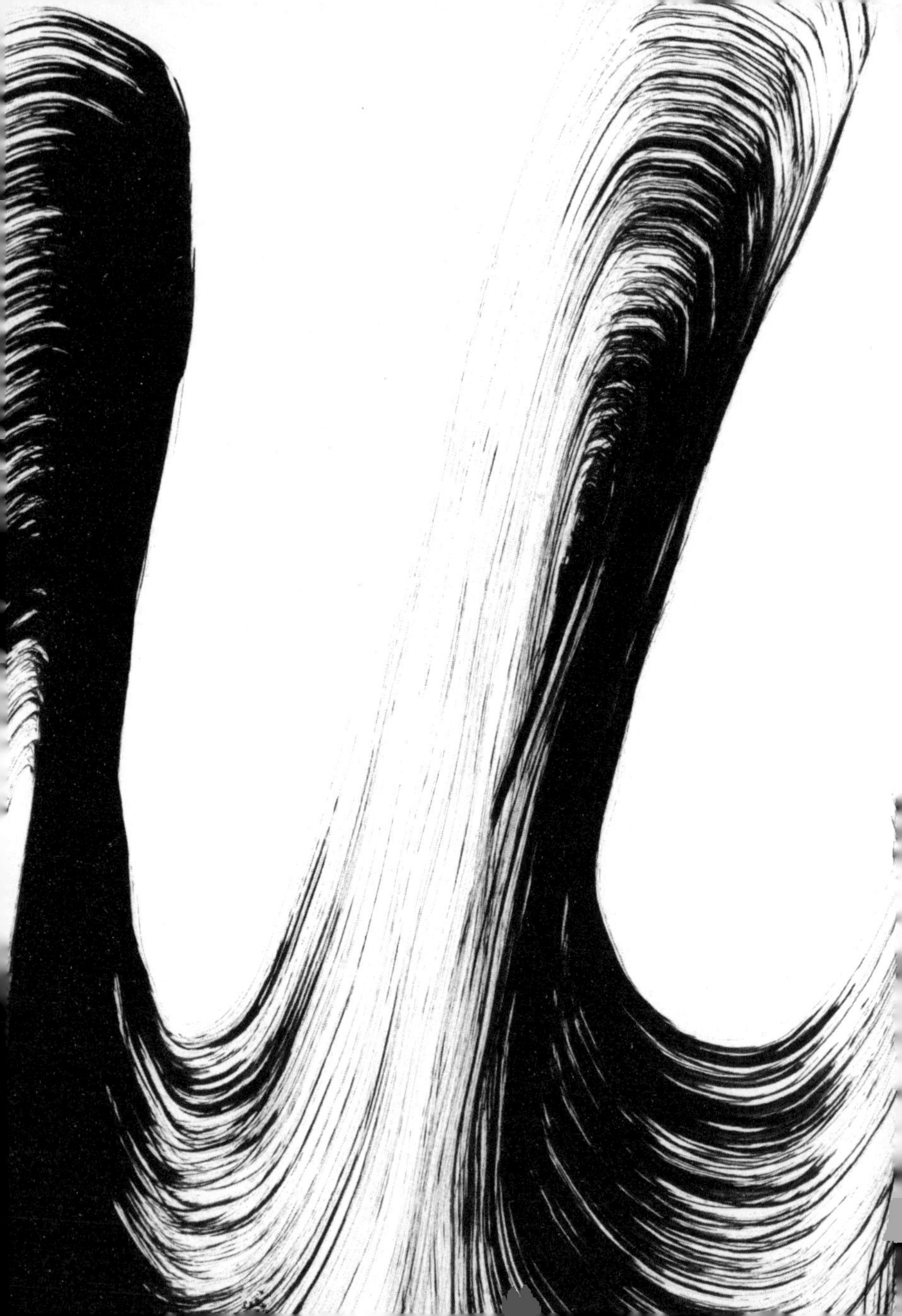

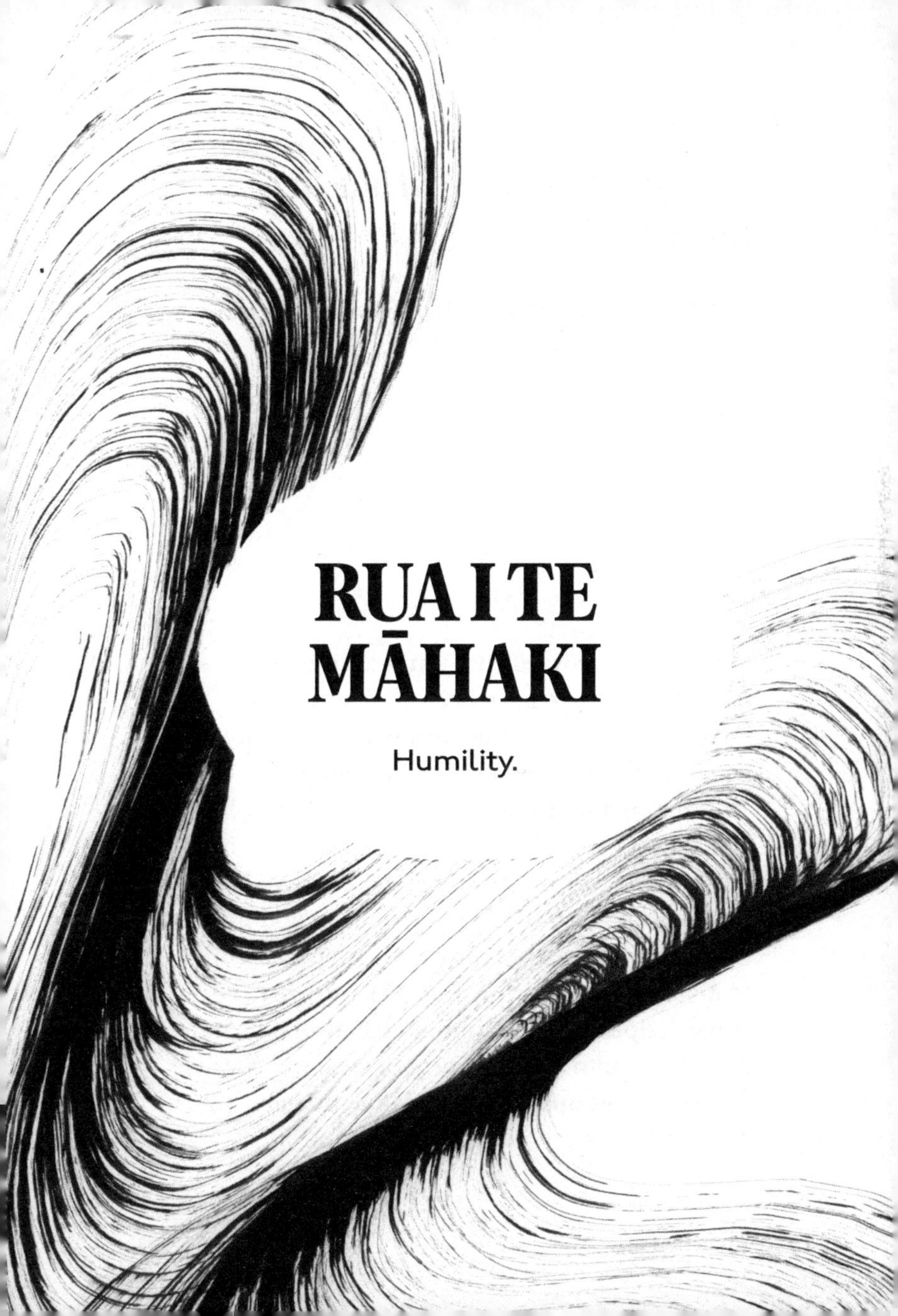

RUA I TE MĀHAKI

Humility.

E kore te kūmara e kī ake he māngaro ia.

The kūmara does not speak of its own sweetness.

Moving ever onwards, we enter a calm and peaceful cave. We have been well prepared by recent lessons on the journey. Thoroughly emotionally cleansed and revitalised in Te Whatumanawa; we reflected in rua i te whai whakaaro; we held the white stone Hukatai in our mouths, helping us to embed the search for knowledge; and we reviewed trust and then immersed ourselves in prayer. The special gifts of matakite, followed by Rehutai, our wise red stone, helped us in beginning to consolidate our knowledge into an awareness of wisdom. Now we find ourselves opening our ngākau māhaki, our humble hearts.

Humility is a central aspect of Hinengaro's ride. This is such a key part of her lesson. Humility is freedom from pride and arrogance, lacking pretence, an openness to face our flaws and mistakes. Humility recognises connection with others and the planet. We are no more important than anyone else. There is a sense of balance to humility.

We see a wide flat stone in the centre of the cave. This is something many of us recognise. It comes from a place called Te Kao in Muriwhenua, named after the process of drying kūmara. Here is a place where our delicious source of sustenance provides the inspiration for thinking about letting go of pride and arrogance.

Rongo, our deity of peace, oversees kūmara cultivation and we can feel his influence. Tensions drift away. We feel settled and open. Growing kūmara was an essential skill for our tūpuna and remains so for many of our communities. Cooked kūmara was traditionally used to take us from a tapu, sacred state to a noa state of normality. Kūmara, simply boiled, is one of those home foods of childhood. Served with just butter and a little black pepper, creating a blissful haven on the tongue and in the puku. The ultimate comfort food.

The kūmara works well as a metaphor when I'm listening to anyone who is lacking in confidence or struggling to find their way. At the right time I have learned to give the example of how kūmara looks a bit lumpy and knobbly, sometimes with fine hair roots sticking out at strange angles, bits of scarred skin, dried grime lingering on the surface. We can all relate! Our feelings are similarly misshapen, our lives messy. And the kūmara is a vegetable that doesn't shout about the delicious taste or its history of sacred skills in removing tapu. In fact, let's be honest, kūmara doesn't look very inviting at all. But when it is boiled, baked, roasted, dried or grilled it is transformed. Moreish, lick-the-lips nourishing tenderness. Our taste buds and our stomachs are so gratified and at peace — a reminder that we are like kūmara. We have a divine centre. Going through the fires of life, our struggles and chaos give us the certainty to be unapologetic about who we are. It helps to remember that without the application of some form of heat, kūmara is hard as a rock and inedible. Through Hinengaro's rua journey, down into the flames of Te Whatumanawa and back again, we are learning by our mistakes, we are listening, we are more open, and we feel an increasing freedom to simply be ourselves. In this way we find our way to ngākau māhaki.

How will you plant your virtual kūmara garden, fertile with humility? How will you tend that garden and pay heed to Rongo's instructions? Maybe you can create an actual kūmara garden and experience the sweetness of sharing the bounty of your labours with your local community. And of course, the extra special joy of eating kūmara that you and your whānau have grown. How can you bring these stories of the kūmara into your whānau? You may be lucky enough to have more stories depending on where you are from. How could you exercise your humility in learning and growing as a kūmara in human form?

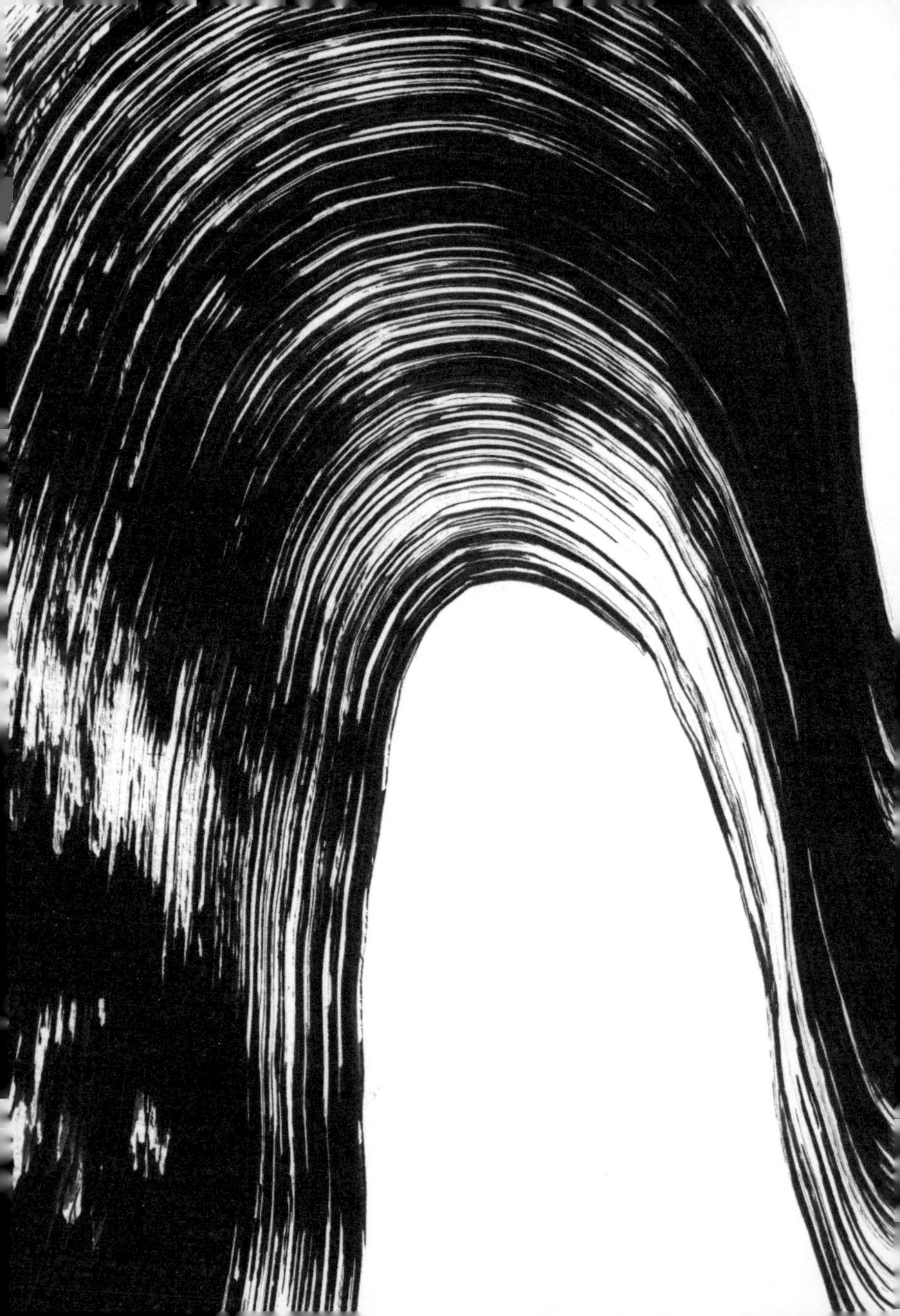

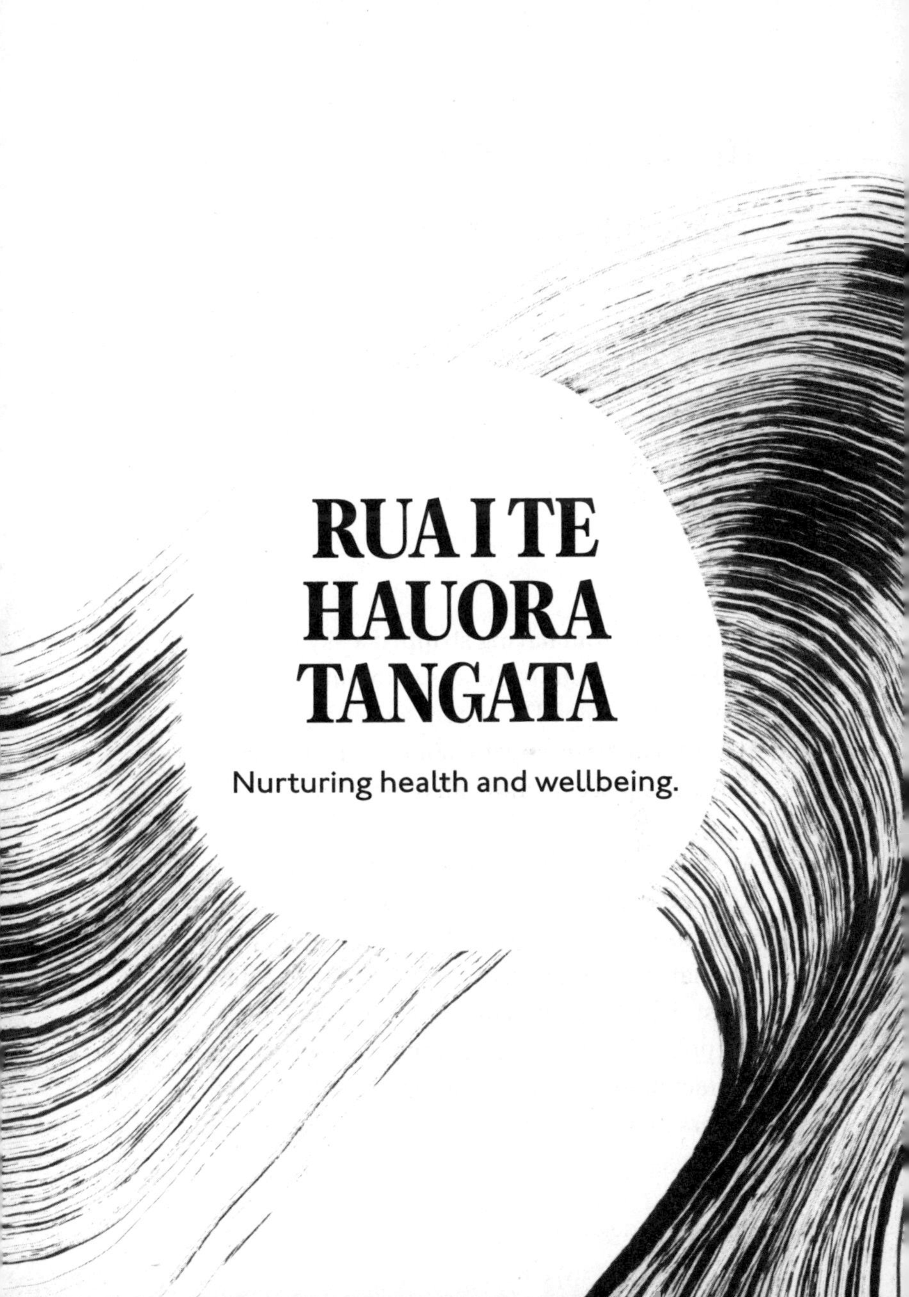

RUA I TE HAUORA TANGATA

Nurturing health and wellbeing.

He kai kei aku ringa.

The results are in our hands.

We emerge from having stripped away our pride and embraced our openness with humble kūmara-filled hearts. Now Hinengaro welcomes us to step into another upper chamber, rua i te hauora tangata, a place to ignite all of health and wellbeing.

An intriguing amber glow welcomes us in. Resinous shapes resembling interlocking starfish greet us at the entrance. Their orange inner glow emanates from the walls around us. We cannot resist. Reaching out a hand, our fingers meet the polished surface of the tentacles, this simple contact unexpectedly warming the palm. Our five fingers map onto these strange, fossilised shapes.

An exchange of energy. This is Hinengaro's entry into her sacred rua i te hauora tangata. Five flaming torches mounted on high around the cave give the illusion of light coming from within the walls themselves. Mahuika's legacy — Takonui, Takoroa, Māpere, Manawa and Tōiti — stand sentinel. Our goddess of fire's children are our witnesses.

We walk forward into a concave space, a scooped-out centre with a dome above. Hinengaro invites us into the palm of her hand.

Ringa, hand, is a word we use as a metaphor for our many roles in life. For example, 'anei te ringa tango otaota', here is the person who pulls the weeds, the person who can triage what is most important and doesn't get distracted by irrelevance. 'Ehara, ko koe te ringa e huti punga ana', 'Indeed, you are the hand that pulls the anchor', meaning you've got this, you have the strength. Anchors back in the day were very heavy stones. 'He ringa whiti' is a person ready to fire up, someone who can go from zero to one hundred in a split second. Ringa hora, a generous individual or group. 'Moea te ringa raupā', marry the one with calloused hands, an industrious person. Ringa wera is the name for those in the kitchen, the cooks with their hot busy hands. Ringa whero, red hand, indicates a chief. And famously, the proverbial saying 'he kai kei aku ringa', literally the food is in our hands: we have the resources, we have the power and skills, we can solve our own problems.

In Muriwhenua we have a saying, 'me tokotoru tātou', 'we are three kinds of people'. Our characteristics are described according to our three types of hands, three types of contributions to the overall wellbeing of our community, our strengths in the ways we take care of the hauora of our people.

Our ringa kaha are the people who make things happen, who ensure all the elements are in place. Sleeves rolled up, reliable, honest, and open. Unwavering problem-solvers. Often unforgiving of those who don't deliver on promises. These are our conscientious and solid hands. The ones who stick it out until the job is done, they always find a way.

Our ringa hāpai or ringa pōpōa are our spiritual leaders. Our hēpara o te kāhui, our shepherds. Theirs are the caring hands that lift our spirits, inspire us with hope, carrying in their hands the unquenchable ability to bring harmony and peace to our lives. They remind us of our intimate connections with the universe.

Thirdly, our ringa ārahi are our visionary leaders. These are the hands that hold us accountable to future generations. Pointing to the health and wellbeing of our descendants. Our ringa ārahi lead by example. Our shining stars, lighting our pathways into the future. Driving us forward with their passion, intellect and wisdom. The hands that gather everyone up and take us forward together.

We all have unique strengths in each of these areas. We all come from whānau, from extended families, with specific traits. Characteristics handed on from generations gone by. We call those shared whānau habits and attitudes 'momo'. Learning from parents and grandparents, we develop with strengths as ringa kaha, ringa hāpai, or ringa ārahi. And we see how certain features come to the fore at different times across the life span. We see our mokopuna dedicated in their wanting to help and contribute to whānau life. Maybe they love to try their hand at sweeping with the broom, to dig in the garden, to be involved in the tasks at home and school, and on the marae.

Our rangatahi, young people, have a natural drive to challenge authority and the status quo. They have a keen eye on the future and their place in it. Our young parents with their go-to attitude of trying again and again, pushing through exhaustion and harnessing their creative ingenuity to meet the needs of our tamariki mokopuna. Our adults and kaumātua have their own spiritual leadership traits. Along with ageing hands, we gain a breadth of perspective that accompanies wrinkles and age spots. Together with all our attributes, our specialties in uplifting the health and wellbeing of others, we nurture each other and ourselves. We can experience the immediacy of our own contribution through our own hands.

Hinengaro takes me to stories of gumdiggers, our ringa kaha of old. These are our forebears who worked hard, often with hand-made tools, to dig kauri gum buried under swamps for export to make resins. This was how many of our tūpuna made a living in the late 1800s and early 1900s. Backbreaking, relentless work. Suffering in harsh conditions. Those ringa kaha are a source of inspiration to us in Muriwhenua. There were ringa hāpai of that era too. Those who encouraged consideration of a deeper meaning despite the hardship. Ringa ārahi were those who worked tirelessly to uphold plans for a better future for generations to come. Our gumdiggers and their communities continue to give us the strength to see ourselves as ringa kaha, ringa hāpai and ringa ārahi.

Hinengaro collects the many life stories of our kaumātua here in rua i te hauora tangata. In this way she continues to give us lived examples of how we can activate our health and wellbeing that go beyond mere words. She gives us these examples to compel us to be sure to discover our own practical resources to inspire holistic health and wellbeing.

Can you see your hands and the hands of your forebears in a new way? What gifts have your tūpuna passed on to you? Maybe you see yourself as a ringa kaha? Or a ringa ārahi or ringa hāpai? These groupings might help to give your aspirations some structure and a sense of purpose for your own role, how to play your part in the health and wellbeing of your whānau. Have a closer look at your own hands: what stories do they tell? What potential for health and wellbeing do you see carved there? What healing traits are handed down from the past that you carry with you into the future? How can you begin to see into those former generations of hands that are part of who you are? How can we use the power that is in our own hands to make this world a better place? We have everything we need to solve our own challenges. How can we truly examine the inspiration in our own hands and then take action?

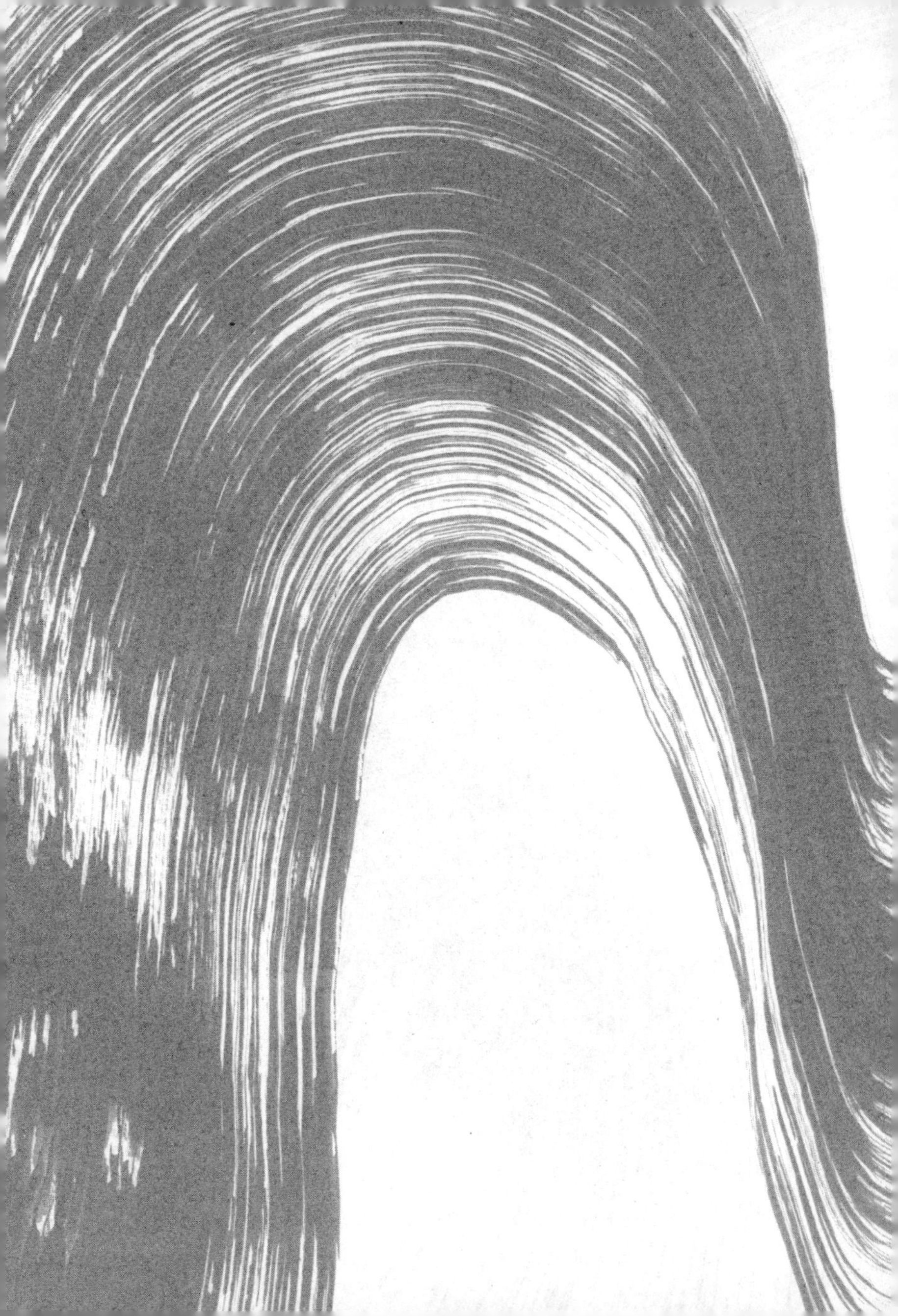

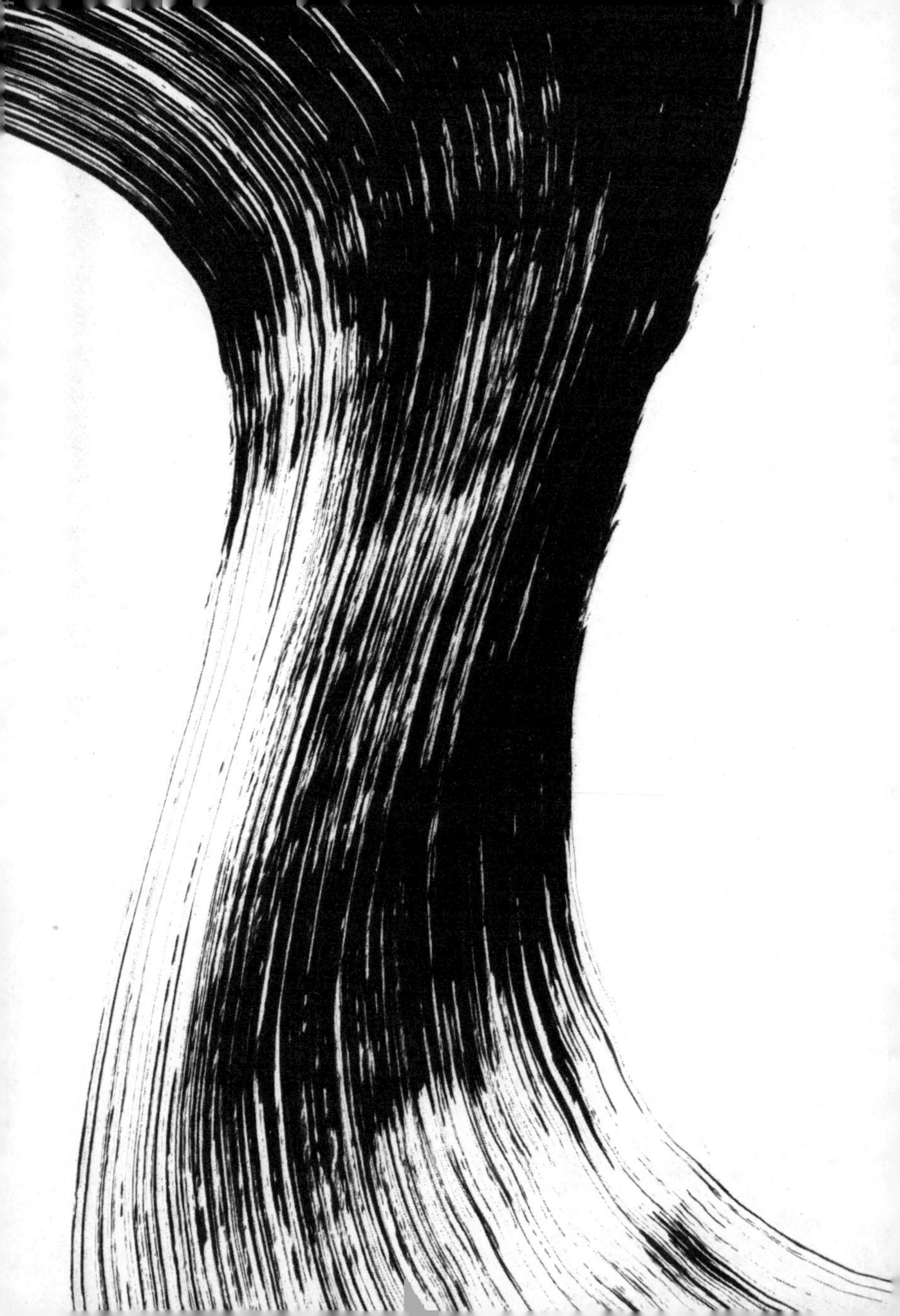

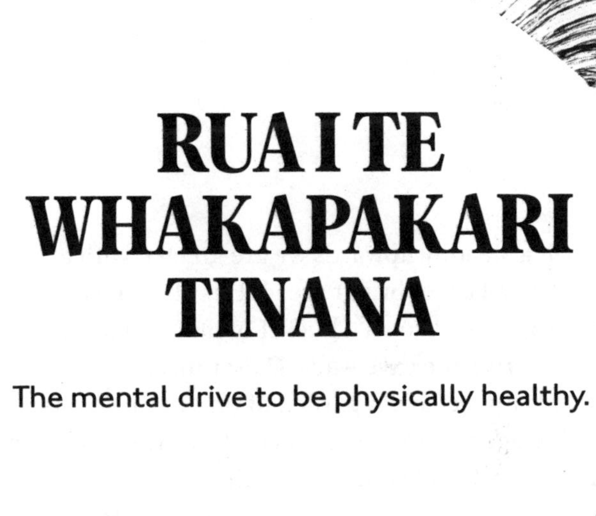

RUA I TE WHAKAPAKARI TINANA

The mental drive to be physically healthy.

Kia uru kahikatea te tū.

Optimal physical growth requires mindful nourishment.

Moving steadily upwards we are greeted with a sudden splash of bright green. It is almost as if someone has thrown a bucket of mint-coloured paint across the cave walls. Closer inspection reveals a spectacular garden of tiny green shoots prying open cracks in the rocks everywhere we look. A rock garden of verdant growth.

We have arrived at the storehouse of strengthening our physical selves with the power of the mind. Here we are tasked with purposeful examination of how our mental capacities influence our bodies' growth. Hinengaro simplifies this for us. She lives in the whole body, not only in the brain. It is

Hinengaro who gives us heart pangs. She is the one who stirs butterflies in our stomachs.

How does rua i te whakapakari tinana begin to take shape for you? Did you experience a bit of heart sink at the thought of focusing on our bodies? Maybe your gut began churning. Perhaps a snowstorm flurry of thoughts and feelings about all the things you chastise yourself about, in not doing enough to look after your body? Feelings of not being good enough, thoughts of being a failure and the repeating frustration every time you consider your relationship with your physical form.

This cave gives us the freedom to shift our entire mindset. I feel myself flying high to stand on the peak of Maunga Piko, the mountain shaped like a newborn fern frond. Maunga Piko, a beacon of growth and potential. A constant reminder of possibility. Hinengaro can transport us from the cave to the mountain top in an instant. Contrast and comparison is something Hinengaro likes to tease us with. She enables us to hold these ideas, feelings, memories, our resistance to change and our hopes, all at the same time.

The matrix of our physical health, all of those

complex concepts and emotions, this fusion of processing comes from Hinengaro.

Seeds of connection have been planted in our mind caves, without us even thinking about it. And that can be alarming: these ideas appearing without our deliberately choosing them. Shaped and brought into consciousness by Hinengaro. She continues to weave our entire web-like history of thought–feeling connections. Here she exposes the apparent separation between thoughts, feelings and our physical selves as false. Hinengaro shows these threads merging into a richer combined experience of who we are. We can't help ourselves, our resolve to manifest more wellbeing in our physical selves begins to unfold.

In contrast to conventional thinking, Hinengaro shows us that body and mind are not separate, even though we speak as if they are. Our ancestors knew it too. The mind–body split problem is something that has been imposed on us in everyday life. We know this separation is not real. We don't live with mind and body as separate experiences. It is only after we are carefully taught to do so that we compartmentalise, literally, these two key parts of who we are.

It's easy to find tangible examples of how far these ideas go in positioning aspects of mind and body as distinct. It can be seen clearly when working in mental health services. For one thing, our workplaces are often tucked away down the back of the hospital campus, in dingy old buildings that are the last to get refurbished. Our departments, our contracting, our service development and delivery are often separate from those related to the physical. People suffering from mental illness over there, those afflicted with physical conditions over here. People with mental illness continue to be stigmatised and blamed for their conditions. Children who are not nurtured emotionally, which often goes unrecognised, suffer from problems with their physical growth and development for the rest of their lives. The separation of concepts of mind and body is not neutral: it perpetuates suffering.

Our Indigenous knowledge systems are holistic woven nets, unfurling strengths across the tides of life. The ancient net expands to catch us when we are struggling. This is in stark contrast to conventional approaches where concepts of illness favour attention to pathology, deficits and shortcomings. How we identify problems and potential is clouded by our model of mind and body. Identifying what is wrong is not sufficient to determine the remedy. We run the risk of labelling people with their illness as a form of identity which becomes internalised and believed. Mind–body separation risks an unnecessary fatalism: people believe they are their illness and this identity is hard to shift once it takes root.

Hinengaro gives us this dedicated rua to conceptualise, determine and decide on our different ways to embrace the needs of our whole being. She paints this picture so vividly for us via the lively growth of plants around these walls. In that way she illustrates that our physical growth comes with an all-encompassing mindset. She reminds us that while we might focus on elements of body and mind, these are interwoven, intimately part of a holistic experience of being. Hinengaro enables our reflection on the progression of mind and body development here in rua i te whakapakari tinana.

Our invitation is to let growth, let the expansion of who we are becoming, do its thing. How can we find a way to trust that the results of that growth will become evident at the right time? Letting our minds move our bodies in healthy ways might take a bit of a leap of faith. But if you think about it, that's what we do instinctively anyway, isn't it?

We get signs, tohu pai, that our minds' efforts are taking effect. We might adjust our posture when we notice we are uncomfortable. Think about how when we are in the garden or outside getting some air, we lift our faces to bathe in the winter sun. Even the idea of doing something, of dancing, can make us smile. We notice thoughts about attraction and feeling sexually aroused and how our bodies respond to these thoughts. We can take time to pay attention to imperceptible movements within us, movements of blood and breath. Pulse and heartbeat. The sensuous brush of skin on our clothes. All of these signals originate with Hinengaro.

Our thoughts can also give us some degree of patience, a chance to observe these changes and to begin to revel in them. We can ease into it and truly appreciate how Hinengaro works from both inside and outside the body.

Rua i te whakapakari tinana is also about ensuring the free flow of mind energy throughout the body, ensuring we don't get stuck in our heads. The flow of mental energy can feel trapped or get blocked, building up pressure, and that risks some sort of blow-out. Maybe we fear losing control and so we hold on tight to our mental stresses and strains. But that logic is flawed. Hinengaro needs to flow through us and the tinana, the body, plays a key role there.

This is often the missing piece when we consider the mind–body interface. Having a regular physical practice that allows mind energy to flow outwards and mitigate any build-ups, blockages or locking up that must burst out eventually. That way we allow a healthy release of pent-up emotions and at the same time provide a chance to shift into a more joyful sense of physical comfort and ease.

Hinengaro's endeavours are emerging, maybe slowly at first. Enjoy the suspense. Relish a deeper awareness of Hinengaro living freely in our whole bodies. Every breath and heartbeat is a chance for our mind–body–wairua system to shift slightly and to realise something we hadn't thought of in quite the same way before. Allow this illumination to intensify. Held in the embrace of this lush cave full of choices and expertise, enjoy a new perspective of the power of Hinengaro in your experience of your body. Be prepared, being in this rua will have you waking up in the middle of the night with new revelations. Let rua i te whakapakari tinana move you in a new direction.

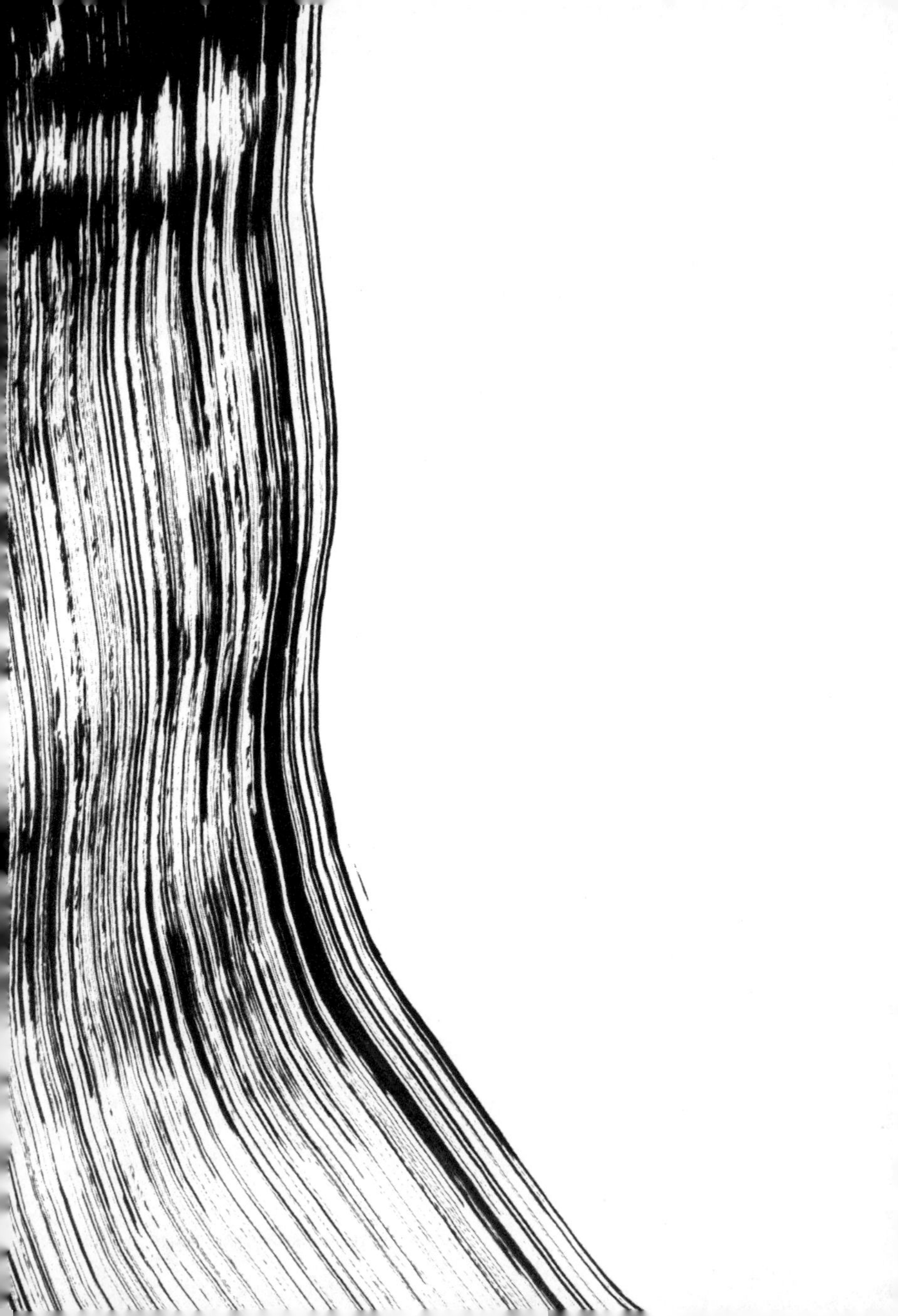

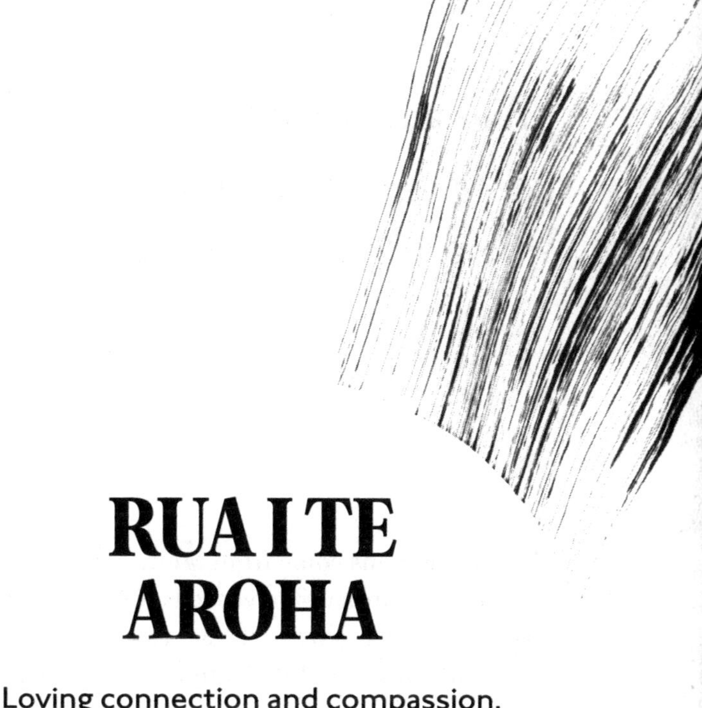

RUA I TE AROHA

Loving connection and compassion.

Aroha atu, aroha mai.

Love given is love returned. Love is a reciprocal energy.

My aroha lessons come from Mum. When I enter rua i te aroha I know she is waiting for me. Together our tears weave a vast cloak. Our falling tears transform into tiny feathers and we add them one by one. Thousands of our daily moments are stitched into the cloak, passed down to her from her mother and her mother and all of our mothers going back to time immemorial. Here is the place where our gossamer-like tendrils of aroha are revitalised in vibrant living colour. That is the magic Hinengaro conjures up for us.

Aroha is an ancient Māori word and concept, describing a deeply felt emotion and a way of thinking that encompasses love, compassion, sympathy and empathy. We consider aroha something that comes from within our core *and* from all around us. An inexhaustible source, a divine wellspring. Aroha is about all the shades of love turning up in our lives. Fierce protection, rage at injustice, smouldering passion and desire, the abyss of loss and grief. I have spent a lot of time in this rua. I have come to the conclusion that a central source of how we experience aroha comes from our experiences of the deaths of those we love and the aroha we carry forward as their legacy.

We have recently left the lush growth of rua i te whakapakari tinana, strengthening our mind–body connections. We have looked more closely at the resourcefulness in our own hands. We have reflected on humility, ngākau mahaki; the red stone of wisdom, and our intuition in rua i te matakite is not far behind. Here, penetrating the rocks, tree roots provide evidence that we are almost at the end of Hinengaro's adventures inside our own mind-caves. Symbols of the origins of our own aroha nourishing the lofty trees above us from down below. We are almost back at the surface.

Entering rua i te aroha, we move through hanging sheets of the most delicate silky gauze. Filaments of lichen-lace form layers of the softest veils, dangling from on high. Light is muted through these shy, loosely draped sheets. We brush through the mycelium curtains, finding our way to a bubbling central pool. Let's put our feet in and feel the sweet relief.

Aroha is our way of expressing what we feel when loved ones pass on. I can still remember when Mum died, even though it was more than 30 years ago. Our mother didn't have a tangihanga, a traditional funeral. She had given her body to the medical school and we received her back a year later in a small box of ashes. That's what she wanted, that was her expression of aroha.

We had a small service for her. I read her favourite poem. Afterwards two women dressed in black came over to our home. They had travelled from Te Kao to pay respects to Mum. We cried. I was pregnant with our son. It was a day of overwhelming aroha-terror. And at the same time aroha whispered about Mum's loving hope for our babies. Aroha can be a tangled muddle. The aroha gasp of what felt like a chasm opening up underfoot. Aroha teaching me how to live, falling through the layers of the loss of our mother. Our whakapapa bridge. The sharp undeniable reality of moving up a generation. Beginning to recognise with a fresh appreciation the way Mum had always held us in so much aroha, bringing us to safety, showing us the way. Now, she guided from beyond the veil. We had to learn new skills to follow her lead, our shared aroha forever in our hearts, in our dreams. Mum would often send us signs at dawn. As eyelids sense light and birds stir.

Experiencing my mother's passing has been such a profound aroha lesson. A lesson that keeps on giving, because that is what aroha does. Aroha seeks to continue to open us up to all the thoughts and feelings that Hinengaro has been hoarding right here to help us recognise how precious life is.

Aroha is how we experience life. Because we are living so close to death.

What do we learn from rua i te aroha? Hinengaro provides a greater appreciation of how precious life is through aroha, and our own aroha legacy is made more pointed in the context and finality of death.

Let's rest here a while. Let our tired feet soak in the warm mineral pool, feeling that aroha bubbling up through our legs all the way to the top of our heads. The steam rising, lifting some of our pain up to be sent through the roots of the mighty trees and away into the wide open realm of Ranginui, our sky father. Aroha is always available. How can we reclaim our aroha birthright? How can we learn the aroha lessons we have been gifted by the passing of our loved ones? How can aroha spur us on to live our lives, honouring the aroha of those who have gone before and those who are yet to be born?

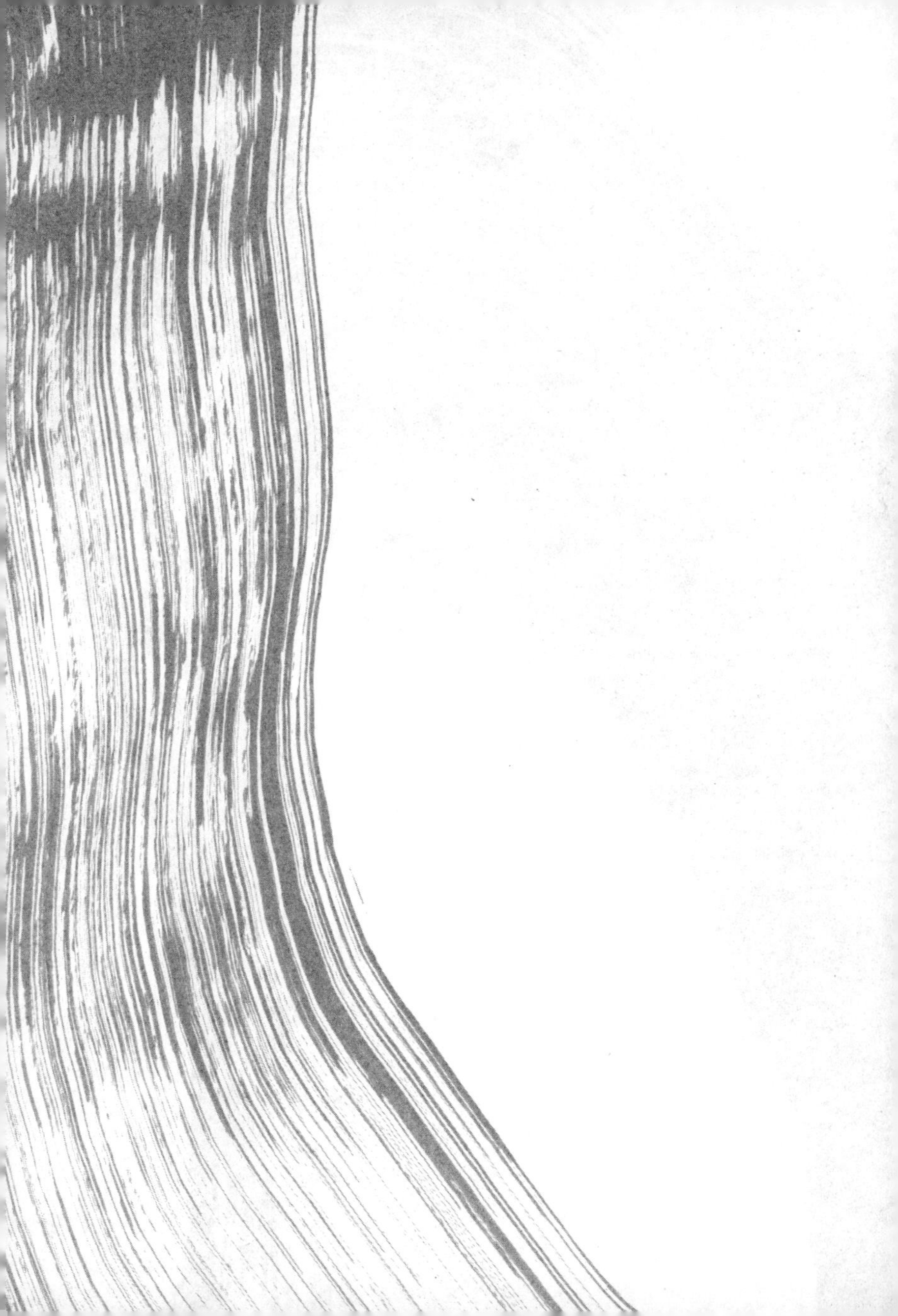

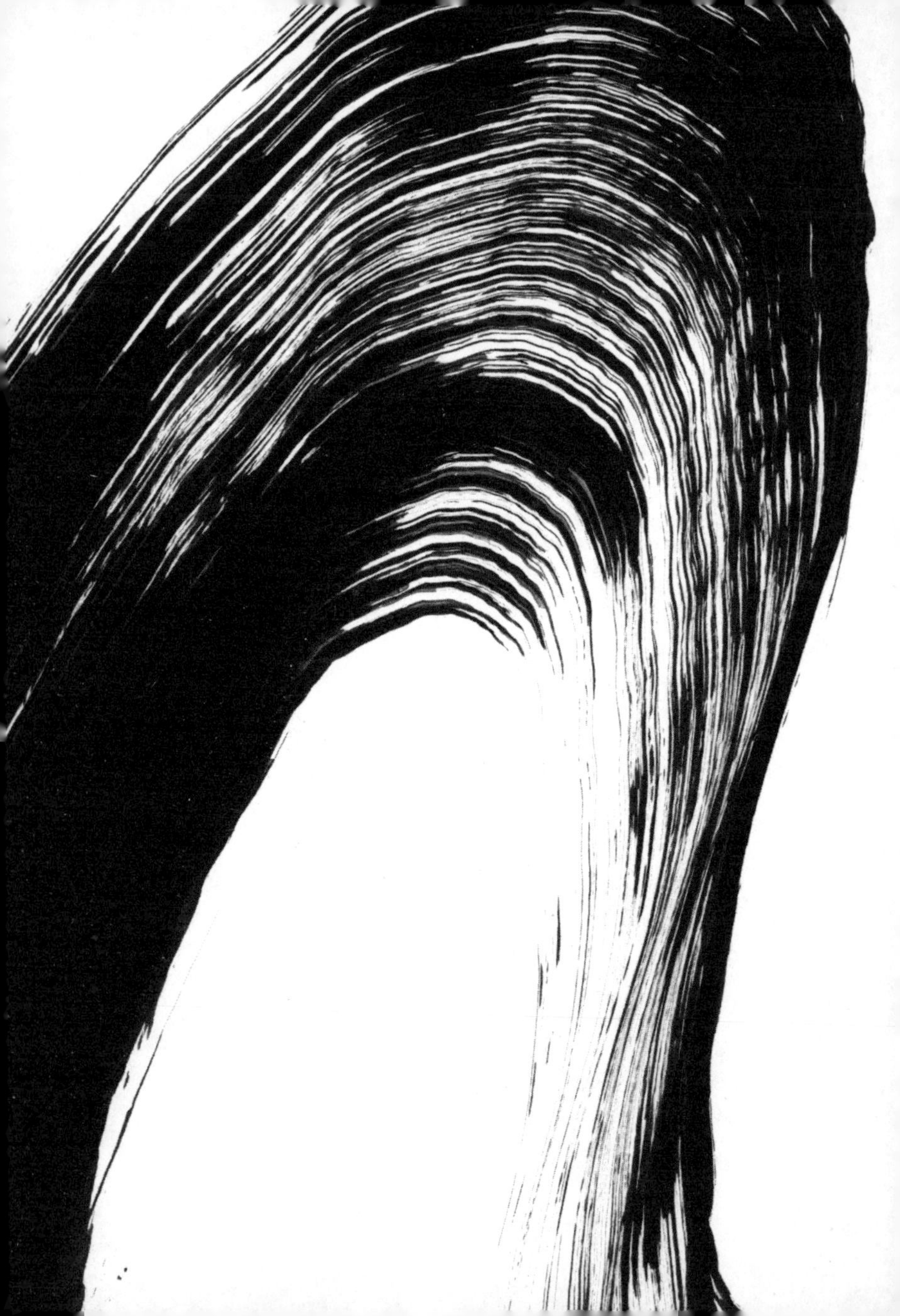

RUA I TE ĀTA WHAKAARO

Deep thought.

Me āta whakaaro ki te tangi o te pūpū harakeke.

Consider the call of the flax snail.

Hinengaro leads us up a series of stony steps to our last refuge, rua i te āta whakaaro. Our eyes become accustomed to the light at the entrance. Elegant leaf spears are silhouetted as our eyes adjust to a vibrant pā harakeke garden in the distance. We are rested, our feet soaked in the restorative rua i te aroha waters. Our hearts awakened by the aroha legacy of loss we share. The aroha effect remains strong.

We see the remnants of a fire nestled in a central stone pit. Embers glowing, sticks at the ready to stoke the flames back to their full glory. Elongated pūpū harakeke shells are scattered around the fire.

For us in the north, especially in Muriwhenua, pūpū harakeke, or pūpū kōrari, flax snails, are a taonga, precious treasures. Pūpū whakarongotauā is another one of their names. The snail that hears the war party. In the past they provided a natural warning system for the local communities. When anyone attempted a stealthy approach, the pūpū would make peculiar sounds. Some accounts emphasise the whistling sound they made as the snails sharply withdrew into their shells. Others recount the sound of them being crushed underfoot by the enemy.

Deep thought, deep reflection. This is Hinengaro's closing priority. Slow down and ponder the lessons from our caving trip through ngā rua a Hinengaro. This kind of contemplation is not always something we make time or space for. Not something we might feel too comfortable about. And yet this is an essential aspect of our wellbeing. This last rua is here for a reason.

Hinengaro has made this our final cave on purpose. How we choose to use the resources of the rua i te āta whakaaro is up to us. How do you feel about the idea of diving deep into your thoughts? Hinengaro has already established that thoughts, feelings, our body, and our spiritual and relational lives are all interwoven and their complex interactions are not usefully considered as solely distinct and separate.

Deep thought is also associated for us with the term 'noho puku', literally, sitting in the stomach. Our puku are symbolically and biologically important places for processing of many kinds. And then for providing the nourishment we need to grow and flourish.

Hinengaro has provided this last cavern in her system to review where we have been and what we have been offered so we can again consider new insights and reflections. Here is a chance to sit back and see this journey as a whole, forming one great complex of learning opportunities for fresh ways to approach life on re-entry back into our lives. A chance to gather up our highlights perhaps. The rediscovery of our stories, our imaginative new perspectives invigorated by Hinengaro.

Picking up the shards of pūpū harakeke shell, we notice some are orange and brown, some are pale cream. Their inner structures are exposed, revealing a miniature version of our journey through ngā rua a Hinengaro. The double spiral of takarangi is here, we can see the miniature stops along the way in the skeleton of our precious pūpū harakeke. The cochlear-like synergy is not lost on us. The clues are evident. We can hold this talisman and rewind our journey.

Hinengaro starts us back at the beginning to summarise all the new ways we are thinking about thinking.

Rewinding back to our entry point, **rua i te horahora**, we began with the generous expanse of spiritual connections, essential for setting ourselves up for success. This is a great reminder to always start from this place of vast interlinking abundance at the beginning of how we prepare for meetings, whānau discussion, and for our own private work on ourselves.

The thrill in learning came next in **rua i te wanawana**. The tingle we feel when we meet our passions in life, and give ourselves the freedom to pursue this drive. Rua i te wanawana fuels the way we pay attention to the juice of learning in all areas of our lives.

Rua i te pūkenga, a focus on shared abilities that we are growing together, was our next stop. Hinengaro points out that this is such a vital priority. When we join up our skills, we are more than the sum of our parts.

The sweet fragrances that trigger memories in **rua i te mahara** were next; Hinengaro has this special place for connecting with the power of memory. Hinengaro reminded us to foster our memory gifts with learning and laughter.

Rua i te pupuke reminded us about patience in building our strengths over time and how that feels emotionally.

The simplicity and stability of **rua taketake o Io** is a formal recognition of the footsteps we follow and those we create for others.

Rua i te atamai demanded our quickest mind-reflexes. Unexpected events mean quick thinking; brevity and some healthy wit are of critical importance in our lives.

This led on to a specific cave for the parenting mind, **rua matua taketake o Tāne**. Caregiving roles are the toughest roles we can ever have. Here is a place to absorb all of Hinengaro's dedicated resources.

Rua i te whaihanga, creativity our birthright, followed next. Many of us have been told our imaginations are not important or even worthwhile. Hinengaro ensures we remember that our own inner lightning sparks are part of our healthy lives.

In **rua i te kōrero**, Hinengaro gave us the power of words. Words can instantaneously take us around the world, back in time and into the future, all in the same moment. Here is a place to remember the extraordinary freedom words can bring us.

Rua i te whakaako is where we entered the place of learning and teaching. Blood, sweat and tears flowed as we neared the deepest part of the journey.

Entering **Te Whatumanawa**, the chasm of lava in the bowels of the earth, we got into the blast furnace of our feelings. We reached our base, our remotest depth. Here Hinengaro reminded us we have these powerful emotions which we can face and recognise as part of who we are.

Beginning to move up again, we entered **rua i te whai whakaaro**, a fitting place to review and reassess in order to develop plans that deliver the results we are looking for.

Then, **rua i te whai mātauranga**, where we were reminded that the search for knowledge is another priority. Hinengaro's Hukatai, the white stone, is our sign of the solemnity of our systems of data gathering and understanding.

Trust, enshrined in **rua i te whakapono**, came next. We were invited to pick up Hinengaro's mānuka as a wero, a challenge, in our lives, remembering the responsibilities that come with building trusting relationships.

Curving ever upwards, the power of prayer echoed in the vast hall of **rua i te karakia**. Each of us comes with different histories of prayer and what that means. Here Hinengaro asked us to apply our most reverent practice in counting our blessings and expressing our gratitude as a health priority.

Next we explored **rua i te matakite**, the ancient gateway opening up our awareness of intuition and second sight. Hinengaro reminded us to trust our gut instincts and to respect cultural experiences that we consider gifts.

Rua i te mōhio asked us to begin to take on board the possibility of wisdom. As our perspectives coalesce, Rehutai, the red stone, is there to help us get a sense of what these tiny morsels of wisdom feel like.

We moved on to the place of humility, **rua i te māhaki**. A reminder from Hinengaro to let go of pride and arrogance, to remember our origins. Our kūmara, along with the deity Rongo, help to keep our humble hearts resilient.

Next on our spiral circuit we visited **rua i te hauora tangata**, where resources in enhancing health in people are stored. Hinengaro reminds us that we have all we need in our own hands.

Rua i te whakapakari tinana followed, where Hinengaro provided the lesson that our minds and bodies are not separate. They are intimately intertwined. We need growth in the mind to grow strong and healthy bodies.

Our penultimate rua was that of **aroha**. We were invited to consider the wellspring of aroha which comes from loss, grief and death. From that place of aroha we are filled with the legacy of those who have passed to make the most of our precious lives.

Finally we arrived here: **rua i te āta whakaaro**. Hinengaro has awakened so many insights through her underground experiences, thinking about thinking in new ways as we sit by the fire, safe and warm. Hinengaro asks us to rest here for a while. What a ride!

Still holding on to our shell, we now know this is a key, returning us to Hinengaro's rua at any time. Whenever we see a shell we will be reminded of our ara, this magnificent pathway. Hinengaro smiles. She has revealed her priorities, held in these rua that guided our tūpuna and remain to guide us and those who come after.

We put a small piece of kindling onto Hinengaro's ahikā. The home fires of Hinengaro continue to burn.

The pūpū harakeke whistle to us as we move out into the sunshine. We will return again and again, trekking through Hinengaro's underground spiral staircase, visiting her rua, enlightening our ara, our journeys of life, death and everything in between.

Index

A note on the illustrations

The artwork for *Ara* reimagines the words of Dr Hinemoa Elder as an intimate, hand-painted series of undulating rhythms. The 23 paintings were made directly on printed templates at a 1:1 scale. I used my favourite paintbrush and a high pigment, easy-flow black paint. I meticulously taped out the titles and the edges to protect the text and amplify a sense of craft. It felt authentic to employ a traditional illustration methodology where practice and intention guided every move. Draughtsmanship became a strategy for reflecting on *Ara*'s sentiments, such as being present and working with your mistakes.

Ara is adorned with hair-like threads that appear almost wind whipped. The painterly and plunging gestures intensify as you get closer to the heart of the spiral, Te Whatumanawa. The brush strokes usher you forward from there, curling and rising to the final rua. The illustrations sometimes appear like honing patterns from a shell, or the shadow of a swivelling echo, a train of thought, a gallant shoreline . . . beating hearts, deep breaths . . . You decide.

I would like to acknowledge two key pieces of research. The first is a specific brushed gouache treatment found in *The Children of Rangi and Papa: The Maori story of creation* by Pauline Yearbury, 1976, where the 'hā' or breath of atua is lightly and thinly painted. It creates a whispering line that is both coming and going at once. The second is Ralph Hotere's drawings in *Mihi: Collected poems* by Hone Tuwhare, 1987, where his urgent mark-making brings drama with operatic delivery — not a transliteration of the author's words, but a beautiful transmutation of them.

My artworks are dedicated to Dr Hinemoa Elder, to the limitless potential she sees in us and the grace with which she leads us there.

Jade Townsend
Ngāti Kahungunu, Te Āti Haunui-a-Pāpārangi

Ngā kupu aumihi

Kei ōku hoa, kei te hunga whai oranga e noho ana ki ēnei rua a Hinengaro hei kāinga ruruhau, hei whare tīhoka, hei nohonga āhuru mōwai ki tēnei ara niko, nei a Mihi ka rere ki a koutou.

E tō mātou pāpā, ko Hirini Wikaira, moe mai rā e te rangatira. Ko te pukapuka nei he roimata nōku, tētahi o tō tauira o mua. E te pāpā, kōrua ko Shane Wikaira, ngā maihi o tēnei wharenui, me kore ake kōrua hei tohutohu ki a mātou. E te whāmere, ko Aunty Thelma Munro, ko Hera Clarke, ko Jesamine Wikaira, ko tātou tērā i te tau 2008. Toitū ngā hua o te wānanga raka, ā, ki ēnei puāwaitanga ki te ao, āmua ake nei.

Ki a Monica Harawira, ki tō tātou Hineraukatauri o te kāinga, e mihi ana ahau ki a koe, ko koe tētahi tino kaitiaki mōku, i reira i taua wānanga. Moe mai rā e te korokoro tūī, e rangona ana e tātou ki tō reo wainene i te tātai whetū i te korowai o Ranginui.

E ngā tongarerewa o tōku ngākau, ki a Reuben kōrua ko Millie. Kei a kōrua tahi te mātāpuna hei whakaohooho manawa kai tūtae i a au.

E taku huatahi nō Ngā-rangi-o-ue, anei aku mihi ki a koe ki ngā wānanga tao, mai ngā tini o ngā huatau ki ngā āpiti rētō o Te Whatumanawa.

E te toki o Muriwhenua, e taku rau matatiki o te kī, Peter-Lucas kāore e ārikarika aku mihi ki a koe cousin.

Kei tōku hoa piripoho nō Tauranga Moana, e Joanna, ko koe taku pou whakawhirinaki i tēnei huarahi ki ngā rua a Hinengaro.

E ngā kaiurungi o tēnei waka i te puna manawa whenua, Margaret kōrua ko Olivia, e hoa mā, tēnā rā kōrua ki tā kōrua whakapau kaha ki te kaupapa nei! Kei te ihumanea, Carla, ko koe te mutunga kē mai o te whakanikoniko i āku tuhinga.

E te parehuia o Rongomaiwahine, e te taura whiri a Hinengākau, Jade Townsend, mai ngā wawata o mua, i te whakaaweawe a Hina, ka puta atu āu mahi ki tōna kōmata o te rangi.

E Tākuta Hōhepa, tōku purapura tuawhiti, ko Darryn Joseph, i te mahinga kai a tēnei pukapuka ko koe te kaingaki tōtō kia whakawhanake ai ngā hua reka.

Kei ngā rua kōhā, kei ngā rua kanapu, kei ngā rua nōki i raro iho i ngā puke kōrero i te taha o Como moana, anei aku mihi mutunga kore. E te Principessa della Torre e Tasso, te tuhi mareikura o Villa Serbelloni, e tūohu nei taku mātenga ki a koe. Ki a koutou ngā manu taiko o Bellagio Residency o te Rockefeller Foundation, i aku hīkoinga, i te taha o te tira e kautere ana, ngā mihi nunui ki a koutou. Rere houtupu ana tēnei kuaka hei tautoko i te kaupapa matua, otirā, ko te mahi ngātahi tātou kia whakahaumanu ai i te oranga o tō tātou ao.

He kupu whakatepe māku, i te puna tukanga auahatanga, anei nga rua o Hinengaro, ngā rua a Hinengaro nōki, hei rauemi oranga tonutanga mā tātou katoa.

Other titles by Dr Hinemoa Elder

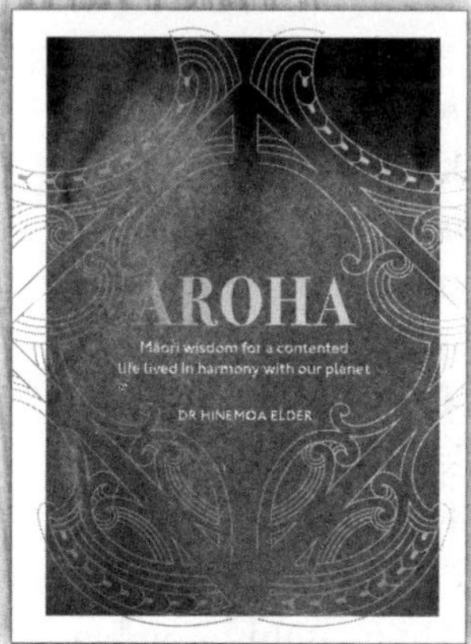

Through 52 whakataukī — traditional Māori life lessons — esteemed psychiatrist Dr Hinemoa Elder shares the power of aroha and explores how it could help all of us every day.

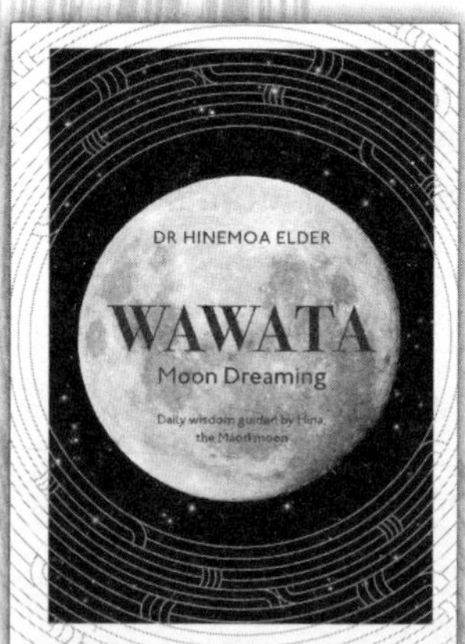

Through the 30 different faces and energies of Hina — the Māori moon goddess — Dr Hinemoa Elder helps to illuminate life's lessons and consider different aspects of life.

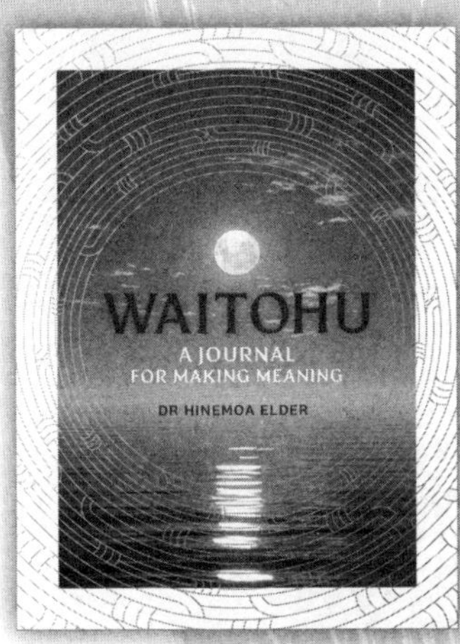

An inspiring journal to record life lessons and help you make deeper connections, guided by Dr Hinemoa Elder's previous books *Aroha* and *Wawata*.

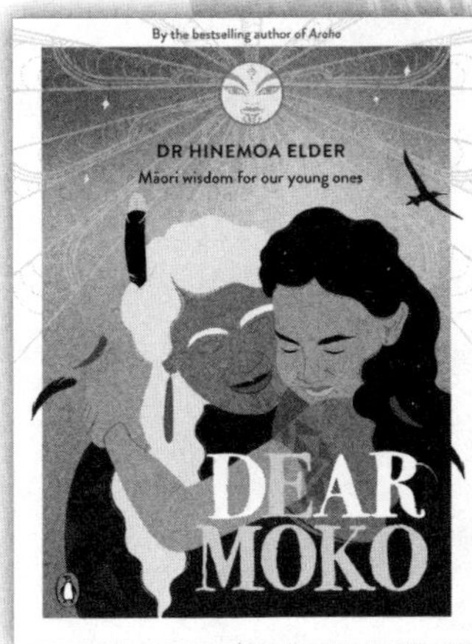

A reshaping of Dr Hinemoa Elder's beloved book *Aroha*, featuring a special collection of whakataukī and whakatauākī for tamariki mokopuna.

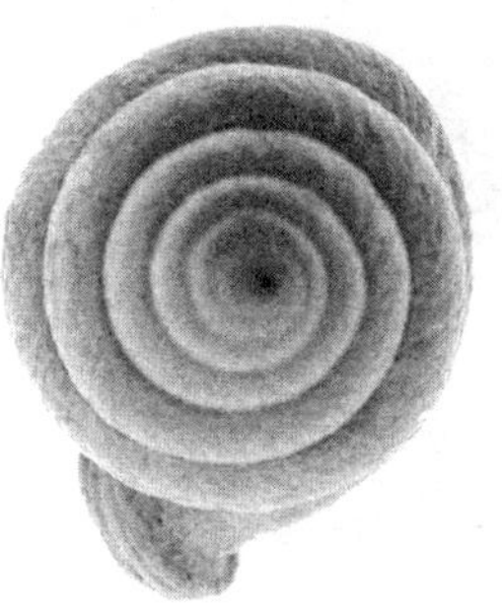

About the author

Dr Hinemoa Elder is of Te Aupōuri, Ngāti Kurī, Te Rarawa, Ngāi Takoto and Ngāpuhi nui tonu descent and is the mother of two adult children.

She has lived on Te Motu Ārai Roa, Waiheke Island for more than 25 years. Hinemoa is the Kaiārahi Oranga Hinengaro at Te Hiku Hauora, Muriwhenua. She also provides youth forensic court reports and neuropsychiatric assessment and treatment for tamariki mokopuna experiencing complexities in their recovery from traumatic brain injury. She is a deputy psychiatry member of the New Zealand Mental Health Review Tribunal.

In 2019, Hinemoa was appointed a Member of the New Zealand Order of Merit for services to psychiatry and Māori. You can find her on Instagram @drhinemoa.

PENGUIN

UK | USA | Canada | Ireland | Australia
India | New Zealand | South Africa | China

Penguin is an imprint of the Penguin Random House group of companies, whose addresses can be found at global.penguinrandomhouse.com

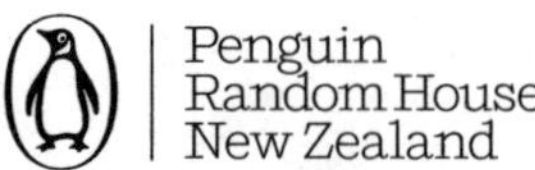

First published by Penguin Random House New Zealand, 2025

Design by Carla Sy © Penguin Random House New Zealand
Illustrations by Jade Townsend
Photographs by Megan van Staden
Printed and bound in China by RR Donnelley

A catalogue record for this book is available from the National Library of New Zealand.

ISBN 978-1-77695-090-4
ISBN 978-1-77695-896-2 (audio)
eISBN 978-1-77695-395-0

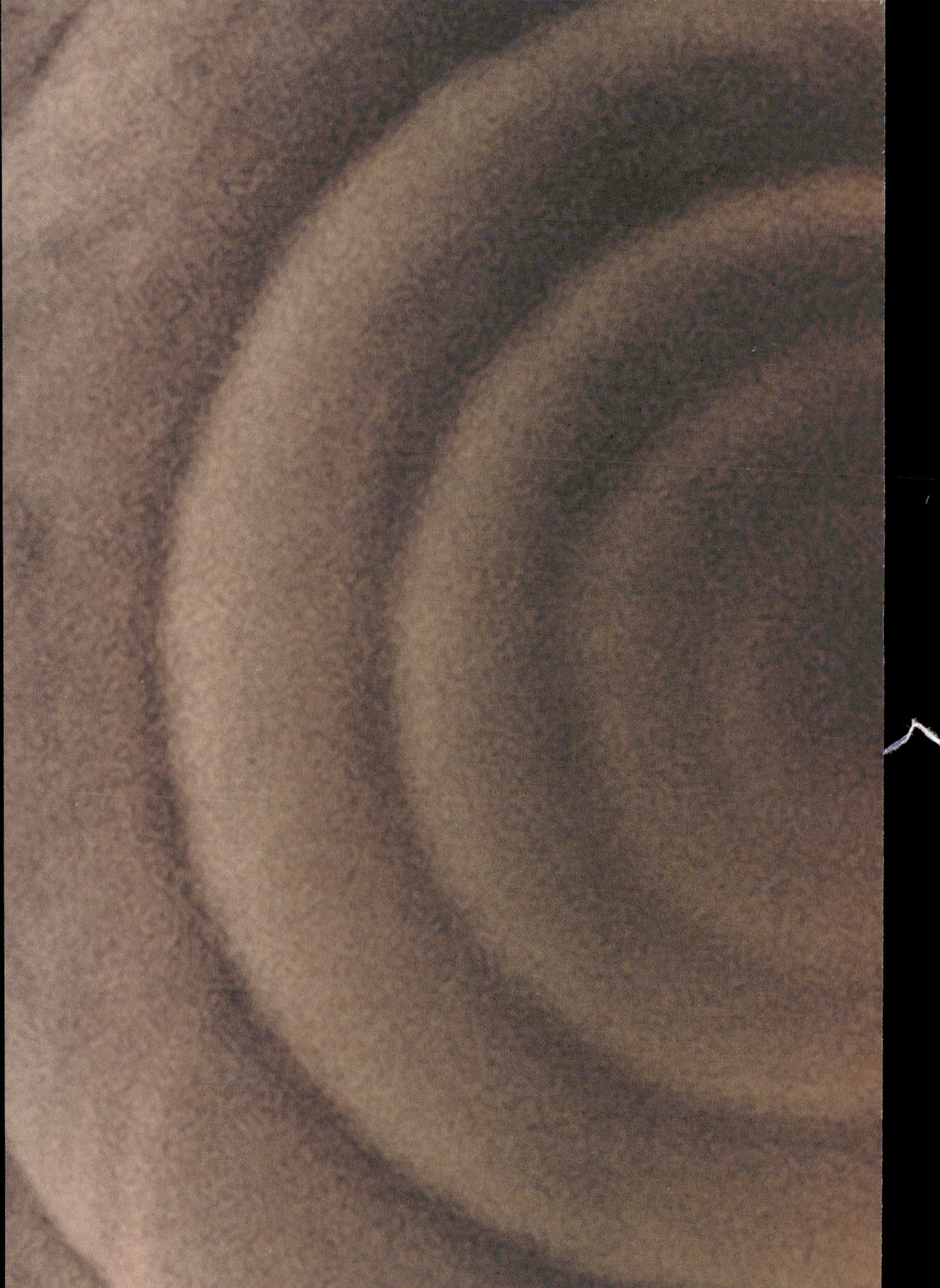